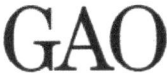
I0415736

June 2012

RYAN WHITE CARE ACT

Improvements Needed in Oversight of Grantees

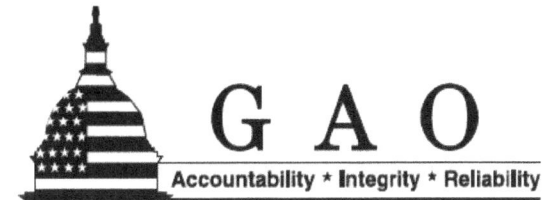

GAO-12-610

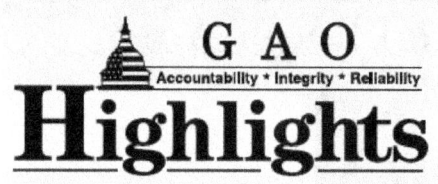

GAO
Accountability * Integrity * Reliability
Highlights

Highlights of GAO-12-610, a report to congressional requesters

RYAN WHITE CARE ACT

Improvements Needed in Oversight of Grantees

Why GAO Did This Study

Each year, half a million people affected by human immunodeficiency virus (HIV) and acquired immunodeficiency syndrome (AIDS) receive services funded by CARE Act grants. HRSA, an agency within HHS, awards CARE Act Part A grants to localities and Part B grants to states and territories. These grantees may provide services themselves or may contract with service providers. HRSA POs monitor grantees, but grantees are to monitor their service providers. PO oversight includes routine monitoring, site visits, and monitoring of special award conditions, such as restrictive drawdown. GAO was asked to 1) evaluate HRSA's oversight of CARE Act grantees and 2) examine steps HRSA has taken to assist CARE Act grantees in monitoring their service providers. GAO conducted a review of grantee files from 2010 and 2011 for 25 selected Part A and B grantees, reviewed HHS and HRSA policies, interviewed HRSA officials, analyzed HRSA data on site visits and interviewed grant officials from GAO's 25 selected grantees and 6 selected service providers.

What GAO Recommends

GAO is making several recommendations, including that HRSA implement key elements of grantee oversight consistent with guidance, including restrictive drawdowns; develop a strategic approach for selecting grantees for site visits; and work to identify grantees' training needs in order to comply with the National Monitoring Standards. HHS concurred with the recommendations.

View GAO-12-610. For more information, contact Marcia Crosse, (202) 512-7114, crossem@gao.gov.

What GAO Found

The Department of Health and Human Services' (HHS) Health Resources and Services Administration (HRSA) does not consistently follow HHS regulations and guidance in its oversight of Ryan White Comprehensive AIDS Resources Emergency Act of 1990 (CARE Act) grantees when conducting key elements of grantee oversight, including routine monitoring and implementing restrictive drawdowns. Additionally, HRSA did not demonstrate a risk-based strategy for selecting grantees for site visits. Project officers (POs) do not consistently document routine monitoring or follow up on that monitoring to help grantees address problems, as required by HHS and HRSA guidance. The purpose of routine monitoring is to enable POs to answer grantee questions about program requirements, provide technical assistance (TA), and follow up on grantee corrective actions in response to previously provided TA. However, GAO found that most POs did not document routine monitoring calls with grantees—only 4 of the 25 PO files GAO reviewed from 2010 and 8 of the 25 files GAO reviewed from 2011 contained documentation of monitoring calls at least quarterly. HRSA often did not follow HHS regulations and guidance in implementing restrictive drawdowns, a special award condition HRSA can place on grantees with serious problems. Restrictive drawdown requires that prior to spending any grant funds, grantees must submit a request, along with documentation of the need, for funds for HRSA review. Six of the 52 Part A grantees and 13 of the 59 Part B grantees were placed on restrictive drawdown from 2008 through 2011. GAO found that HRSA did not consistently provide grantees in GAO's sample that were on restrictive drawdown with the reasons the restrictive drawdown was implemented, instructions for meeting the conditions of the restrictive drawdown, or guidance on the types of corrective actions needed. This has limited the effectiveness of restrictive drawdown as a tool for improving grantee performance. Regarding the oversight of grantees through site visits, HRSA did not demonstrate a clear strategy for selecting the grantees it visited from 2008 through 2011. For example, HRSA did not appear to prioritize site visits to grantees based on the amount of time that had passed since a grantee's last site visit. Although many HRSA POs GAO spoke with said that site visits were a valuable and effective form of oversight, GAO found that 44 percent of all grantees did not receive a site visit from 2008 through 2011 while others received multiple visits.

Grantees are required to oversee the service providers with whom they contract and in April 2011, HRSA issued the National Monitoring Standards for grantee monitoring of service providers. The standards describe program and financial requirements and include 133 requirements for Part A grantees and 154 requirements for Part B grantees. Though the standards were intended to improve grantee monitoring of service providers, some grantees said that a lack of training and TA has hindered its implementation. Additionally, some grantees have found the requirement for annual site visits of service providers to be challenging. HRSA officials said that they believe they provided adequate training to grantees in implementing the standards, which did not represent new requirements.

Contents

Abbreviations

ADAP	AIDS Drug Assistance Program
AIDS	acquired immunodeficiency syndrome
CARE Act	Ryan White Comprehensive AIDS Resources Emergency Act
DFI	Division of Financial Integrity
EHB	electronic handbook
EMA	eligible metropolitan area
HAB	HIV/AIDS Bureau
HHS	Department of Health and Human Services
HIV	human immunodeficiency virus
HRSA	Health Resources and Services Administration
MAI	Minority AIDS Initiative
NARA	National Archives and Records Administration
NASTAD	National Alliance of State and Territorial AIDS Directors
NOA	notice of award
OMB	Office of Management and Budget
PO	project officer
TA	technical assistance
TGA	transitional grant area

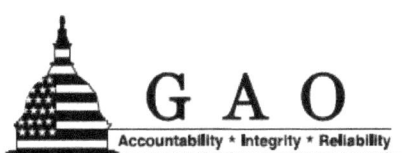

United States Government Accountability Office
Washington, DC 20548

June 11, 2012

The Honorable Tom Harkin
Chairman
The Honorable Michael Enzi
Ranking Member
Committee on Health, Education, Labor and Pensions
United States Senate

The Honorable Richard Burr
Ranking Member
Subcommittee on Children and Families
Committee on Health, Education, Labor and Pensions
United States Senate

The Honorable Tom Coburn
Ranking Member
Permanent Subcommittee on Investigations
Committee on Homeland Security and Governmental Affairs
United States Senate

An estimated 1.2 million people in the United States are living with human immunodeficiency virus (HIV) infection in 2012, and approximately 50,000 new infections occur annually. Since the first cases of acquired immunodeficiency syndrome (AIDS) were reported in June 1981, more than 600,000 people with AIDS have died. Each year, half a million uninsured or underinsured individuals and families affected by HIV/AIDS receive assistance funded by grants provided for in the Ryan White Comprehensive AIDS Resources Emergency Act of 1990 (CARE Act).[1] CARE Act funds are distributed to grantees such as states, localities, and other public or nonprofit entities; these grantees may provide CARE Act program services themselves or may contract with service providers to

---

[1] Pub. L. No. 101-381, 104 Stat. 576 (codified, as amended, at 42 U.S.C. §§ 300ff through 300ff-121). The 1990 CARE Act added title XXVI to the Public Health Service Act. Unless otherwise indicated, references to the CARE Act refer to current title XXVI. The CARE Act programs have been reauthorized by the Ryan White CARE Act Amendments of 1996 (Pub. L. No. 104-146, 110 Stat. 1346), the Ryan White CARE Act Amendments of 2000 (Pub. L. No. 106-345, 114 Stat. 1319), the Ryan White HIV/AIDS Treatment Modernization Act of 2006 (Pub. L. No. 109-415, 120 Stat. 2767), and the Ryan White HIV/AIDS Treatment Extension Act of 2009 (Pub. L. No. 111-87, 123 Stat. 2885).

offer the medical care or support services needed to achieve positive medical outcomes.[2] The CARE Act is administered by the Department of Health and Human Services' (HHS) Health Resources and Services Administration (HRSA). In fiscal year 2012, HRSA allocated over $2.3 billion of its annual appropriation to CARE Act programs.

Members of Congress have asked questions about HRSA's ability to adequately oversee Ryan White grantees and service providers to ensure that CARE Act funds are used properly and effectively. CARE Act grantees are monitored by HRSA project officers (PO) and other grants management officials, and federal regulations require grantees to monitor their service providers' compliance with program requirements. Grantees or service providers found to be in violation of program or federal grants management requirements are to receive technical assistance (TA) or other corrective actions designed to bring them into compliance.[3] In this report, we (1) evaluate how HRSA oversees CARE Act grantees and (2) examine steps HRSA has taken to assist CARE Act grantees in monitoring their service providers.

There are five primary parts (Parts A through D and Part F) of the CARE Act under which HRSA awards grants. The types of entities eligible for grants and types of services provided through the grants vary by part. In fiscal year 2011, the majority of CARE Act grants are awarded under Parts A and B. Part A grants are awarded to the eligible metropolitan areas (EMAs) and transitional grant areas (TGAs) most severely affected by the HIV/AIDS epidemic and comprise about 30 percent of CARE Act grants.[4] Part B grants are awarded to states, the District of Columbia, and

---

[2]We use the term "grantees" to refer to organizations or entities that receive funding directly from HRSA for CARE Act services, and the term "service providers" to refer to organizations awarded contracts or subgrants from grantees to provide services or arrange for another organization to provide services. Grantees may also provide services themselves.

[3]HRSA defines technical assistance as the delivery of practical program and technical support which may include necessary technical and nonfinancial assistance, fiscal and program management assistance, operational and administrative support, and the provision of information to grantees regarding the variety of resources available to them, and how those resources can best be used to meet the health needs of their clients.

[4]EMAs are areas that have a population of 50,000 persons or more and had a cumulative total of more than 2,000 new AIDS cases during the most recent 5-year period. TGAs are areas that have a population of 50,000 persons or more and had a cumulative total of 1,000 to 1,999 new AIDS cases during the most recent 5-year period.

U.S. territories and associated jurisdictions and comprise about 55 percent of CARE Act grants. Part B also provides for grants under the AIDS Drug Assistance Program (ADAP) through which drugs are provided to eligible individuals with HIV/AIDS.[5] Our review was limited to Part A and Part B grantees and their service providers.

To evaluate how HRSA oversees CARE Act grantees, we reviewed HHS and HRSA policies and procedures, conducted a review of selected grantee files, interviewed selected Part A and Part B grantees, HRSA POs, and selected national organizations with HIV/AIDS expertise, and reviewed HRSA data on site visits and staffing. First, we reviewed HHS and HRSA policies and procedures for overseeing grantees and service providers. We interviewed HRSA staff about policies and procedures for overseeing grantees and service providers, as well as about coordination among HRSA oversight personnel. Second, we selected a nongeneralizable sample of 25 of the 111 Part A and Part B grantees—12 of the 52 Part A grantees and 13 of the 59 Part B grantees.[6] To select our sample we divided all of the Part A and Part B grantees into two categories based on whether or not they had been found to be in violation of program or financial requirements from 2008 through 2011. We then chose grantees from each of these two categories to reflect a range of funding levels, geographic factors, and grant longevity. We reviewed the files HRSA maintained for this nongeneralizable sample of 25 Part A and Part B grantees. We reviewed these files for grant years 2010 and 2011.[7]

---

[5]Title XXVI of the Public Health Service Act contains several parts which provide for grants for various HIV/AIDS-related services. In addition to Parts A and B, Part C provides for grants directly to public and private nonprofit entities to provide early intervention services; Part D provides for grants to organizations for family-centered medical and support services for women, infants, children, and youth with HIV/AIDS and their families—including infected and affected family members; and Part F provides for grants for demonstration and evaluation of models of quick response HIV/AIDS services and electronic data systems, training of health care providers, and the Minority AIDS Initiative (MAI). Part E does not provide for funding for HIV/AIDS Services but rather includes provisions to address various administrative functions.

[6]The selected Part A grantees were Baltimore, Maryland; Baton Rouge, Louisiana; Denver, Colorado; Detroit, Michigan; Indianapolis, Indiana; Las Vegas, Nevada; Memphis, Tennessee; New York, New York; Phoenix, Arizona; St. Louis, Missouri; San Francisco, California; and West Palm Beach, Florida. The selected Part B grantees were California, Florida, Georgia, Louisiana, Maryland, Mississippi, Nebraska, New York, Nevada, Ohio, Pennsylvania, Rhode Island, and South Carolina.

[7]The grant year for Part A is from March 1 through February 28. The Part B grant year is from April 1 through March 31.

Our file review included a review of the grantees' reports for grant years 2010 and 2011 in response to requirements, located in HRSA's Electronic Handbook (EHB); review of external audit files for these grant years; and review of the grantee's PO files, which include important documentation of site visits and routine monitoring, among other things, for these grant years. To conduct this file review, we developed and used a data collection instrument to determine if the files included evidence of required monitoring and key monitoring documents. Third, we conducted structured interviews with POs that had responsibility for monitoring grantees selected for our file review about the grantee files, and obtained their views on their roles and responsibilities and on HRSA's policies and procedures.[8] We also conducted structured interviews with all 25 of the grantees selected for our file review to learn about how HRSA oversees its grantees. In addition, we interviewed staff from national organizations with HIV/AIDS expertise, including the Kaiser Family Foundation, the National Alliance of State and Territorial AIDS Directors (NASTAD), the Communities Advocating Emergency AIDS Relief Coalition, the ADAP Advocacy Association, and the National Association of County and City Health Officials. Fourth, we analyzed data provided by HRSA on its oversight of grantees, including PO staffing and HRSA site visits.[9] To assess the reliability of these data we compared the data provided to us by HRSA with information provided to us by our selected 25 grantees when possible. We asked HRSA to resolve discrepancies either within the data or between the data and information provided by our selected grantees. We generally found all of the data reliable for our purposes. We also assessed HRSA grantee monitoring processes described in documentary and testimonial evidence against relevant criteria, including HHS policies, HRSA policies, Office of Management and Budget (OMB) guidelines, and federal regulations for grants management.[10]

---

[8] Within HRSA, POs from the HAB Division of Service Systems are responsible for the oversight of Part A and B grantees. For purposes of this report, when we refer to HRSA POs, we are referring to POs within that division.

[9] For the purposes of this report, we assessed HRSA site visits that included the grantee's PO or other HRSA staff. HRSA refers to these types of site visits as comprehensive site visits and these visits are central to the agency's routine monitoring of grantees. We did not assess other types of site visits.

[10] CARE Act grants are subject to governmentwide uniform administrative requirements for grants and cooperative agreements which for HHS are codified in title 45 of the Code of Federal Regulations. In this report, these requirements are referred to as "federal regulations."

To examine steps HRSA has taken to assist CARE Act grantees in monitoring their service providers, we conducted interviews of grantees and service providers, interviewed HRSA staff, and reviewed HRSA standards. First, we conducted structured interviews with all 25 of the grantees selected for our file review and a nongeneralizable sample of 6 service providers to learn about how grantees monitor their service providers. We included only those service providers that provide medical services.[11] We selected our sample of 6 service providers based on the grantees' responses to our questions about frequency of service provider site visits, the frequency and type of TA they provide to their service providers. HRSA provided us with a spreadsheet listing all of the service providers for each of our 25 grantees. We limited this list to service providers that received at least $100,000 in CARE Act funding and provided medical services.[12] We then selected one service provider from this limited list for each of 6 grantees using the information indicated above. Second, we interviewed HRSA staff about policies and procedures for overseeing grantees and service providers. Third, we reviewed the HRSA National Monitoring Standards, which were developed by HRSA to help Part A and Part B grantees meet federal requirements for program and financial monitoring of their service providers. These standards were implemented in 2011.

We conducted this performance audit from April 2011 to June 2012 in accordance with generally accepted government auditing standards. Those standards require that we plan and perform the audit to obtain sufficient, appropriate evidence to provide a reasonable basis for our

---

[11]We selected service providers from Indianapolis, Indiana; New York, New York; and Phoenix, Arizona. We also selected service providers from Florida, Pennsylvania, and Rhode Island.

[12]HRSA categorizes service providers by four broad service types—administrative service, medical service, support service, and HIV counseling and testing. Administrative services are those related to grants management and monitoring activities including the development of management systems and preparation of reports. Medical services are those outpatient and ambulatory care services that are part of essential medical care. They can include, for example, oral health care and HIV/AIDS drug assistance. Support services are nonmedical services tied to medical outcomes. They can include, for example, client transportation to medical appointments and substance abuse residential services. HIV counseling and testing includes the provision of voluntary HIV testing to help people learn their HIV status. We excluded service providers that provided only HIV counseling and testing, administrative services, and/or support services. Service providers that provide medical services in addition to any of the excluded services were included in our selection.

findings and conclusions based on our audit objectives. We believe that the evidence obtained provides a reasonable basis for our findings and conclusions based on our audit objectives.

Background

Under the CARE Act, Part A and Part B grantees are awarded grants to provide a range of services—both medical and support—to uninsured and underinsured clients with HIV/AIDS. In fiscal year 2011, most CARE Act funding was distributed to grantees either as base or supplemental grants. Base grants are distributed by formula, which includes a grantee's share of living HIV/AIDS cases.[13] Supplemental grants are generally awarded through a competitive process based on the demonstration of severe need and other criteria. Part A provides for grants to EMAs and TGAs. EMA and TGA funding is primarily provided through three categories of grants: (1) formula grants, (2) supplemental grants, and (3) Minority AIDS Initiative (MAI) grants.[14] Part B provides for grants to states, the District of Columbia, and U.S. territories and associated jurisdictions. These grants include (1) formula grants, (2) supplemental grants, (3) ADAP formula grants,[15] (4) ADAP

---

[13]Part A and Part B formula grants are based on reported living HIV/AIDS cases as of December 31 in the most recent calendar year for which data are available.

[14]MAI grants are supplemental grants awarded on a competitive basis to address disparities in access, treatment, care, and health outcomes.

[15]Through ADAP grants, medications are provided for the treatment of HIV disease. Congress typically designates a portion of the Part B appropriation for ADAP each year. A formula based on the number of reported living HIV/AIDS cases in the most recent calendar year is used to award ADAP formula funds to states, the District of Columbia, and territories and associated jurisdictions. Additionally, 5 percent of the ADAP appropriation is to be reserved for supplemental grants to states and territories that have demonstrated severe need. ADAP funds may also be used to purchase health insurance for eligible clients covering medications and primary care services as long as the cost does not exceed the cost of otherwise providing ADAP medications covered by the program.

supplemental grants,[16] (5) MAI grants, and (6) supplemental grants for states with "emerging communities".[17,18] Part A and Part B grantees apply for funding annually.[19]

The PO is the HRSA official responsible for working with grantees in overseeing the programmatic and technical aspects of the Part A and Part B grants. Within HRSA, POs in the HIV/AIDS Bureau's (HAB) Division of Service Systems are responsible for the oversight of Part A and Part B grantees. POs are supervised by HAB Division of Service Systems branch chiefs, who are responsible for ensuring that POs are meeting their oversight responsibilities.[20] The PO works with the HRSA Office of Financial Assistance Management's grants management specialists (GMS). GMSs are responsible for providing nonprogrammatic administrative assistance to grantees, including assistance in interpreting provisions of grants administration, law, regulation and policy. These provisions include how grantees can draw down grant funds and how grantees are to administer and close out grants. GMSs are supervised by Grants Management Officers. Additionally, within the Office of Federal Assistance Management, staff in the Division of Financial Integrity (DFI) provide TA and advice to the POs and GMSs.

---

[16]HRSA awarded $50 million in both 2011 and 2012 for ADAP emergency relief funding in order to address states' increased need for medications for CARE Act clients.

[17]"Emerging communities" are defined as metropolitan areas reporting between 500 and 999 cumulative AIDS cases over the most recent 5 years.

[18]The CARE Act provides that Part A and B base and supplemental grant funds are available for obligation by the grantee for a 1-year period beginning on the first day of the grant year. It also requires HRSA to cancel any unobligated balances at the end of the grant year, recover funds that had been disbursed to grantees, and redistribute these funds to grantees in need as supplemental grants. Grantees must estimate their unobligated balances during the grant year and provide final amounts in their federal financial report. Grantees may request to carryover funds for 1 additional grant year. See GAO-09-984 and GAO-09-1020.

[19]The grant year for Part A is from March 1 through February 28. The Part B grant year is from April 1 through March 31.

[20]Branch chiefs have sometimes been needed to serve as POs for some grantees due to staffing shortages in recent years. According to a HRSA official, serving in these dual roles is difficult and does not allow the time necessary to supervise and develop POs.

HRSA POs conduct their oversight of Part A and Part B grantees in accordance with regulations and guidance. HHS grants management regulations and guidance govern all HHS grants, including CARE Act grants. The regulations and guidance provide for the creation of agency and program-specific guidance. Where HRSA has not created specific guidance, POs and GMS follow the overarching HHS regulation and guidance. Therefore, POs follow HHS regulations and guidance and any additional HRSA-specific grants management guidance when it is available. HRSA officials told us POs are to follow the Division of Service System Operations Manual (HRSA Operations Manual), which provides guidance and protocols specifically for PO oversight of CARE Act Part A and Part B grantees. The HRSA Operations Manual was first provided to us in August 2011 and updated in December 2011.[21] Because the updated HRSA Operations Manual was not in existence during the majority of the period covered by our review, we primarily refer to HHS grants management regulations and guidance in our evaluation of HRSA's oversight. HRSA's grantee oversight includes several elements, described below.

Routine Monitoring

HRSA POs are responsible for overseeing the Part A and Part B programs by conducting routine monitoring of grantees' performance and compliance with statutory requirements, regulations, and guidance. Routine monitoring includes regularly scheduled monitoring calls, reviews of grantee reports, and the provision of TA to grantees. HHS guidance indicates that monitoring activities are to be documented. This guidance also indicates that the documentation is to include information about the type of follow-up actions recommended or taken. We found that POs were assigned an average of six Part A and Part B grantees to oversee at a time. If during the course of routine monitoring a PO finds that a grantee has not met its program or financial requirements, the PO is responsible for determining, in consultation with his or her branch chief, whether a grantee requires more intensive monitoring including a special condition of award, such as restrictive drawdown. The PO is responsible for monitoring any of these special conditions put in place. POs are HRSA's primary contact with Part A and Part B grantees, and they are to communicate with their assigned grantees at least monthly. In addition to

---

[21]The August 2011 version of the HRSA Operations Manual did not include all of the information and policies that were included in the version provided to us in February 2012, which was dated December 2011.

a scheduled routine monitoring conference call with grantee management, POs are to respond to interim grantee e-mails and calls and to provide guidance and TA as needed.

As part of routine monitoring, POs are also responsible for reviewing reports filed by grantees to fulfill HRSA's annual reporting requirements. These reports are intended to help HRSA identify grantee problems with program implementation and ensure grantees' compliance with federal statutes, regulations, and guidelines. In fiscal year 2012, Part A grantees are required to submit 11 different reports while Part B grantees are required to submit 16 reports. The reports contain important programmatic and financial information such as descriptions of funded services, annual expenditures, and grantee accomplishments and challenges in meeting program goals. POs are to provide feedback to grantees based on their review of these reports and provide written requests for changes to reports which are submitted through EHB. The PO and GMS are also responsible for reviewing grantee reports to ensure that grantees are spending funds in accordance with the grant terms and conditions and POs and GMSs are to coordinate in their review of grantees' reports. Grantee reporting requirements are listed in appendix I.

When a PO identifies a problem during routine monitoring the PO is to provide TA to help the grantee understand the changes needed to address the problem. TA is a targeted means of addressing a particular issue or problem and is provided to ensure that program implementation reflects the most recent requirements. The overall intent of TA is to assist the grantee in improving its capacity, effectiveness, and efficiency. A PO may provide the TA by phone, email, on-site or at grantee conferences. POs may provide the TA or assist grantees in obtaining TA from HRSA consultants.[22]

Site Visits

In addition to their overall routine monitoring responsibilities, POs are to participate in site visits for Part A and Part B grantees. Site visits are intended to provide the PO with an opportunity to review the program,

---

[22]HRSA contracts with consultants to provide TA to improve the performance of CARE Act grantees, and to assist them in addressing the HRSA priority areas with the goal of enhancing their performance as grantees. HRSA consultants may also conduct site visits focused on the priority areas. HRSA consultants are not federal employees, and are generally employed by management and/or health services consulting firms.

and may act as a TA session for the grantee. HRSA guidance states that site visits should be viewed as an opportunity to expand on information grantees have provided in their CARE Act grant application, responses to reporting requirements, and conference calls. During a site visit, the PO may meet with grantee and service provider staff to obtain feedback on how the program is functioning, visit various locations at which service providers deliver services, and review grantee and service provider program documentation. For the Part A and Part B programs, HRSA does not have written guidance describing its policy for the selection of grantees to visit; however, agency officials told us that they prioritize site visits based on two elements—grantees without a recent site visit and grantees with problems. In addition, a federal course which HRSA has offered to all of its employees for several years and requires all new POs to take indicates that agencies should determine which grantees to visit based on an analysis of risk, which includes a consideration of grant funding level as an indicator of potential risk, among other things.[23]

When planning a site visit, POs are to provide advance notice in writing to the grantee of the intended site visit along with a copy of the site visit agenda and the tool the PO will be using to evaluate the grantee. The tool addresses the priorities listed below during the site visit. If the site visit will involve the review of a priority item in which the PO does not have specialized training, such as clinical quality management, the PO can consider bringing one or more HRSA consultants for the visit.

According to HRSA guidance, POs are to focus on the following priorities during the grantee site visit (listed below in order of highest to lowest priority):

- assure grantee compliance with CARE Act provisions and HRSA guidance by reviewing compliance with the basic funding requirements, such as the presence of an adequate plan for the use of grant funds and administrative, program, and financial requirements;

---

[23]*Monitoring Grants and Cooperative Agreements for Federal Personnel*, Section 6-1. According to HRSA, the HHS Office of Grants and Acquisition Policy and Accountability worked with a contractor to develop a series of classes on federal grants management. This manual corresponds with one of the classes in that series.

- assure basic functioning of the Part A and Part B programs by reviewing, for example, the grantee's ability to disburse funds to service providers in a timely fashion and the grantee's ability to conduct program and financial monitoring of service providers;

- assure access to care by reviewing the grantee's clinical quality management processes and the grantee's assessment of unmet need for HIV/AIDS services in their jurisdiction;

- assure coordinated systems of care by reviewing the grantee's efforts to coordinate with other CARE Act programs, HIV counseling, testing and prevention programs in their area, and other programs that provide access to HIV/AIDS treatment including Medicaid and Medicare;[24] and

- document and report the impact of the grantees' use of CARE Act funds including any program innovations and/or program successes.

Upon arrival at the site visit location, the PO is to meet with the grantee leadership and the Part A or Part B program staff. During the initial meeting, the PO is to review the intent of the visit and the site visit agenda. This meeting is also an opportunity for the grantee to provide an update on the status of the program and the delivery of services. During the site visit, the PO is to take notes on the priorities listed above, and be prepared to conduct an exit conference with the grantee leadership and program staff to explain both preliminary positive and problem findings. The PO is to prepare a site visit report to document his findings and recommended corrective actions. Additionally, recommendations are to be provided for follow-up TA if appropriate and any special action steps that the PO will take to help the grantee address the site visit findings. HRSA guidance updated during our review states that the site visit report is to be provided to the grantee within 30 days of the visit.

---

[24]Medicaid is the federal-state program that covers acute health care, long-term care, and other services for certain categories of low-income individuals. Medicare is the federal health insurance program for people aged 65 and older, certain individuals with disabilities, and individuals with end stage renal disease.

Single Audits	Part A and Part B grantees are subject to the requirements of the Single Audit Act, as amended, and the act's implementing OMB guidance.[25] These provisions require grantees that expend $500,000 or more in federal awards in a fiscal year to have a single audit for that year conducted by an independent auditor. HRSA's Division of Financial Integrity (DFI) reviews grantees' single audit reports with findings related to CARE Act programs along with corrective action plans provided by the grantee in response to any audit findings.[26] Federal regulations require HRSA to use single audits as a tool to monitor Part A and Part B grantee compliance with program and financial requirements.
Restrictive Drawdown	In accordance with federal regulations, HRSA may impose special restrictive conditions on a grantee's award if HRSA determines that the grantee violated program or financial requirements, or has insufficient management systems or practices to ensure stewardship of grant funds or achievement of award objectives. These issues may be identified through routine monitoring activities, site visits, or single audits. One such condition is called restrictive drawdown.[27] Restrictive drawdown requires that prior to spending any grant funds, grantees must submit a request for funds for HRSA review by the 20th of each month, for the upcoming month, or no less than 10 days before the grantee intends to expend the funds. With each request, the grantee must submit supporting

[25]The Single Audit Act as amended, 31 U.S.C. §§ 7502 et seq., requires states, local governments, and nonprofit organizations expending $500,000 or more in federal awards in a year to obtain an audit in accordance with the requirements set forth in the act. A single audit consists of (1) an audit and opinions on the fair presentation of the financial statements and the Schedule of Expenditures of Federal Awards; (2) gaining an understanding of and testing internal control over financial reporting and the entity's compliance with laws, regulations, and contract or grant provisions that have a direct and material effect on certain federal programs (i.e., the program requirements); and (3) an audit and an opinion on compliance with applicable program requirements for certain federal programs. We refer to these audits as single audits—they are also commonly referred to as A-133 audits. *See* OMB Circular No. A-133.

[26]DFI is responsible for notifying grantees of the adequacy of their proposed corrective actions and for consulting with other HRSA staff, including POs, as needed.

[27]The notice of award (NOA) is the official document that states the terms, conditions, and amount of a grant award and is signed by the official who is authorized to obligate funds on behalf of HRSA. An NOA shows the amount of federal funds available to the grantee and is issued at the start of each grant year. A revised NOA may be issued during a grant year to effect an action resulting in a change in the amount of support or other change in the terms and conditions of award such as a restrictive drawdown.

documentation including all grantee invoices, and other financial documents related to the request.[28] Upon PO review and approval of the request and related documentation, HRSA is to make CARE Act funds available to the grantee. In December 2011, during the course of our review, HRSA created agency-specific guidance that specified the reasons Part A and Part B grantees might be placed on restrictive drawdown, how a grantee is to be notified of this special condition, and under what conditions a grantee can be removed from restrictive drawdown. However, this guidance was not in place during the period covered by our review.

National Monitoring Standards for Grantee Monitoring of Service Providers

Federal regulations require grantees to oversee their service providers. In April 2011 HRSA compiled existing requirements into a comprehensive document called the National Monitoring Standards.[29] The standards are designed to help Part A and Part B grantees meet federal requirements for program and financial management, and to improve program efficiency. Prior to HRSA's issuance of the standards, guidance on how to ensure grantee compliance with program requirements and how to monitor service providers was found in multiple sources. HRSA expects the standards to provide direction to grantees for monitoring their own compliance with CARE Act program and financial requirements and the performance of their service providers.

HRSA officials told us that the national monitoring standards were developed in response to two HHS Office of Inspector General reports that identified the need for a specific standard regarding the frequency and nature of grantee monitoring of service providers and a clear PO role

---

[28]Part A and Part B grantees that are not on restrictive drawdown are able to request funds that they have available at any time during the grant year through the use of an online form that is submitted to the HRSA Payment Management System. Additional documentation is not required. Fund requests are reviewed and upon approval are provided to the grantee the next business day.

[29]HRSA states that the standards are based on administrative requirements for HHS grant awards, Office of Management Budget principles, the HHS Grants Policy Statement, the NOA and Conditions of Award for CARE Act grants, and HRSA program guidance.

in monitoring grantee oversight of service providers.[30] The standards were compiled by HRSA with assistance from a national team of financial and program experts and a working group of Part A and Part B grantees. According to HRSA, the working group provided feedback on drafts of the standards. Additionally, according to HRSA, the standards were presented to all Part A and Part B grantees in a 2010 Grantee Meeting. Grantees were notified of their obligation to comply with these standards in fiscal year 2011.

Grantee Files

HRSA maintains three different grantee files to assist in its provision of oversight, monitoring, and TA to Part A and Part B grantees and there is a different record retention period for each of these three files.[31] Single audit reports and related financial documentation are maintained in hard copy audit files by HRSA's DFI. HRSA's record management program requires these files to be kept onsite at HRSA for at least 2 years after the final close of the audit or upon resolution of any adverse audit findings. The files are then to be sent to the Federal Records Centers to be maintained for an additional 4 years.[32] The EHB includes the NOA and official grantee reports in response to CARE Act grantee reporting requirements listed in appendix I. It is maintained electronically by the HRSA Division of Grants Management Operations and the Division of Service Systems and documents in EHB are accessed by POs and other grants management staff as part of their routine monitoring responsibilities. Currently, HRSA maintains the EHB for 6 years, but is

---

[30]U.S. Department of Health and Human Services Office of Inspector General. "Monitoring of Ryan White CARE Act Title I & II Grantees." (Washington, D.C.: U.S. Government Printing Office, 2004). http://oig.hhs.gov/oei/reports/oei-02-01-00640.pdf and U.S. Department of Health and Human Services Office of Inspector General. "The Ryan White CARE Act Title I & II Grantee's Monitoring of Subgrantees." (Washington, D.C.: U.S. Government Printing Office, 2004). http://oig.hhs.gov/oei/reports/oei-02-01-00641.pdf.

[31]Under the Federal Records Act, agencies are to manage the creation, maintenance, use, and disposition of records in order to achieve adequate and proper documentation of the policies and transactions of the federal government and effective and economical management of agency operations. 44 U.S.C. chapters 21, 29, 31, and 33. Accordingly, to ensure that they have appropriate recordkeeping systems with which to manage and preserve their records, agencies develop records management programs that include, among other things, specified retention periods for agency records.

[32]Federal Records Centers across the United States store and provide access to inactive or permanent records pending their disposition according to the approved records retention periods.

working to finalize a record retention period. Additionally, PO files, which include the only documentation of routine monitoring, site visits, and TA, and duplicate copies of the required grantee reports that are also found in EHB, are maintained in hard copy by the PO. During the course of our review, HRSA officials told us that HRSA's record management program requires these files to be maintained for the current and previous grant year, after which they were to be destroyed.[33] The December 2011 update to HRSA's Operations Manual now suggests that POs should maintain copies of site visit reports for at least 5 years, and that any documents related to issues under investigation not be discarded. However, this change does not apply to other key documentation in PO files, such as regularly scheduled conference calls and copies of relevant e-mails.

HRSA Does Not Consistently Follow Guidance on Oversight of Grantees and Faces Other Challenges

HRSA does not consistently follow HHS or its own guidance for grantee oversight when monitoring CARE Act grantees. A lack of records and frequent changes in PO assignments further challenge HRSA's ability to oversee grantees and to assist them with program implementation.

HRSA Does Not Consistently Follow Applicable Guidance for Grantee Oversight

HRSA did not consistently follow guidance for documenting routine monitoring, prioritizing grantee site visits, reviewing annual single audit findings, or clearly communicating with grantees about the restrictive drawdown process.

HRSA Did Not Consistently Document Routine Monitoring

POs do not consistently document routine monitoring or follow up on that monitoring to help grantees address problems. HHS guidance indicates that monitoring activities performed in order to evaluate grantees' programmatic performance, including any discussions with grantees, should be documented. This guidance also indicates that documentation of monitoring actions is to include information about the type of follow-up actions recommended or taken. However, we found that most of the PO files that we reviewed did not contain documentation of routine monitoring

---

[33]Although HRSA's record management program requires these records to be kept for 2 years, the grantee records made available to us typically included information for less than 2 full grant years.

calls—of the 25 PO files for grantees in our sample, only 4 PO files contained documentation of monitoring calls at least quarterly in the 2010 grant files we reviewed, and only 8 contained documentation of quarterly calls in the 2011 grant files.[34] Though most of the files we reviewed contained documentation of e-mails between POs and grantees indicating that communication was taking place, HRSA POs are to conduct and document regularly scheduled calls. Despite the lack of documentation in PO files, most grantees we interviewed reported having regular communication, via phone or e-mail, with their POs. Seventeen of the 25 grantees confirmed that their PO conducted regularly scheduled conference calls, and 7 noted that these calls included a set agenda.

Most grantees said they had received feedback at least once from a PO on a required report, but eight noted that such feedback was uncommon. Grantees submit numerous reports throughout the year containing important programmatic and financial information. HHS guidance states that monitoring is to include a review of reports, and that review of reports may help officials identify performance or financial issues that require follow-up. Further, HRSA POs are to review and provide feedback and guidance to grantees on program and fiscal reports. However, seven grantees said that feedback on reports was not specific or timely. Only four grantees told us that they received PO comments on their reports during monthly monitoring calls, though HRSA states that reporting requirements are to be discussed during routine calls, which are intended to provide POs with an opportunity to provide such feedback. While a lack of feedback might indicate that a PO had no concerns about a grantee's reports, POs may be missing opportunities to use the information provided in reports to better communicate with grantees about their compliance with program requirements and help grantees make improvements. Seven grantees stated that they would appreciate receiving more feedback on the reports they submit to ensure they were meeting HRSA's standards.

---

[34]Early in our review, HRSA told us that POs were to conduct quarterly conference calls with their grantees. In June 2011, POs were told that they were to contact their grantees monthly using a conference call template covering a set of monitoring topics. Because this change occurred after the start of our review period, we assessed files based on calls at least quarterly. HRSA later told us, however, that POs have always had to conduct and document monthly calls with grantees, but that this was not consistently adhered to prior to June 2011.

Some grantees told us that TA was not helpful because POs sometimes provide conflicting or delayed guidance. TA is a key step toward addressing grantee challenges with program implementation identified during routine monitoring. Though eight grantees described occasions when they received helpful TA from HRSA staff or contractors, eight noted that PO responses to their questions were sometimes delayed or inconsistent with past verbal guidance provided by their current or a past PO, making it difficult for them to understand what changes were needed. For example, one grantee told us it takes an excessive amount of time for their PO to answer their questions, and another said that PO responsiveness varied.

Further, four of the 25 grantees said they were told that HRSA could not provide needed TA due to budget constraints, forcing the grantees to seek TA from other sources or using their own administrative funds. Three of those grantees told us that they hired TA providers using their administrative funds, but one added that the TA cost $30,000 out of their limited administrative budget, which they noted might not be an option for many grantees. The CARE Act requires that grantees spend no more than 10 percent of their grant on administrative activities, which include TA and service provider monitoring activities. Three other grantees told us they turned to NASTAD for TA when HRSA could not provide it or when PO responses to their questions were delayed.[35] Some grantees noted that HRSA had provided assistance through national TA calls and webinars, and one added that calls and webinars were a useful substitute for on-site TA when travel funds are limited. One grantee explained that they received helpful TA from their PO by phone after a planned TA visit by the PO was cancelled by HRSA due to constrained travel funds.

We found that 6 of the 25 grantee files we reviewed from 2010 and just 2 of the 25 files from 2011 contained documentation of TA reports and that few files contained documentation of PO discussions of corrective actions with grantees. HHS guidance states that monitoring activities and any resulting follow-up on identified performance issues must be documented, and issues are to be addressed as soon as possible by providing TA and ensuring grantees take needed corrective actions. Three grantees told us

---

[35]HRSA currently has a 3-year cooperative agreement with NASTAD to provide TA to ADAPs regarding issues including client waiting lists, cost containment, and other financial challenges. NASTAD also maintains a listserv to facilitate peer-to-peer TA between Part B grantees.

that PO follow-up on TA was vague or delayed, though two grantees told us that their POs did conduct follow-up on TA in monthly conference calls. Two grantees told us that though they informed HRSA in writing of their proposed action steps in response to TA recommendations, HRSA did not provide feedback on their proposed corrective actions. Another grantee said that they were unable to address site visit findings due to a lack of timely TA related to the findings.

Some grantees said that their need for TA was exacerbated by the lack of a current program manual. For example, one grantee explained that a manual would help them with matters such as grantee reports. HRSA officials confirmed that the most recent Part A and Part B manuals were issued in 2006, and stated that these printed manuals were not updated to reflect the 2009 CARE Act reauthorization. While HRSA officials stated that policies and procedures had been made available on the CARE Act website, they acknowledged that information for grantees is not available in the form of a comprehensive program manual similar to the printed manual that was last provided in 2006. Seven grantees noted that more written guidance, including an up-to-date electronic program manual, would help them with many of their routine questions or TA needs, which often revolve around questions about CARE Act program requirements. Two grantees added that such written guidance would be especially beneficial for new grantee staff or newer grantees. Further, one of the service providers we spoke with stated that it did not find the HRSA website to be helpful because links were not always kept up to date. The Comptroller General of the United States' Domestic Working Group found that establishing departmentwide policies and procedures on an internet site is beneficial to grantees because it allows grantees to find detailed information in a single location.[36] HRSA officials said that they recently issued a survey to obtain feedback from grantees about HRSA's program operations and processes, including the frequency and timeliness of PO communication with grantees and their satisfaction with TA provided by HRSA through conference calls, the HRSA website, and HRSA

---

[36]The Comptroller General of the United States' Domestic Working Group. *Guide to Opportunities for Improving Grant Accountability* (Washington, D.C.: October 2005). The Domestic Working Group was established in 2001 and is chaired by the Comptroller General of the United States. This group consists of 19 federal, state, and local audit organizations. The purpose of the group is to identify current and emerging challenges of mutual interest and explore opportunities for greater collaboration within the intergovernmental audit community. Providing a guide to address grant accountability was one such challenge.

contractors. They said that they plan to use the results of this survey to improve their interactions with grantees.

HRSA Did Not Prioritize Site Visits Strategically

HRSA did not follow its own policies for selecting the grantees it visited from 2008 through 2011, and varied in its timeliness for providing site visit follow-up. According to HRSA officials, the agency cannot visit all of its 111 Part A and Part B grantees each year due to staff and budget constraints. Therefore, it is necessary for HRSA to be strategic in selecting which grantees to visit in any given year. HRSA does not have written guidance describing its policy for the selection of grantees to visit; however, agency officials told us that they prioritize site visits based on two elements—grantees without a recent site visit and grantees with problems. In addition, the Monitoring Grants and Cooperative Agreements for Federal Personnel manual, which accompanies a federal course which HRSA has offered to its employees for several years and requires all new POs to take suggests that agencies should determine which grantees to visit based on an analysis of risk, which may include the two elements HRSA told us it uses, as well as a consideration of grant funding level, among other things. However, our review of HRSA site visit data suggests that HRSA did not consistently select the grantees it visited based on these three elements.

First, HRSA did not prioritize site visits based on the amount of time that had passed since a grantee's last visit. Specifically, although many HRSA POs we spoke with said that site visits were a valuable and effective form of oversight, we found that 44 percent of all Part A and Part B grantees did not receive a site visit from 2008 through 2011. In addition, 6 of the 25 grantees we interviewed told us that there had been a significant amount of time between HRSA site visits they had received or since their most recent site visit, ranging from 5 to 12 years. One of these grantees said that its first HRSA site visit after 12 years led to the grantee being placed on restrictive drawdown. Grantee officials said that they believed that if HRSA had not waited 12 years to conduct a site visit there would have been far fewer findings because they would have been making necessary adjustments with each periodic site visit. An additional indication that HRSA does not consider time since last visit when scheduling site visits is the fact that HRSA does not maintain a centralized list of site visits that have been conducted. In order to provide data on their site visits for the purpose of our review, HRSA extracted data from travel records. Without centralized site visit data, HRSA would not be able to readily track this element when determining which grantees to visit

Second, HRSA did not always appear to prioritize site visits based on a grantee's history of problems. Based on HRSA data, we found that 30 percent of all Part A and Part B grantees with a history of problems did not receive a single HRSA site visit from 2008 through 2011.[37] In addition, only three of the nine Part A and Part B grantees with the most HRSA site visits from 2008 through 2011 had been placed on restrictive drawdown. While HRSA visited these grantees three or more times, other grantees that were placed on restrictive drawdown received two or fewer HRSA site visits during these 4 years. Although HRSA officials told us that restrictive drawdown is not the only indication of grantee problems, they said they impose it when the grantee has a history of serious problems. We found that some grantees with numerous site visits had not been placed on restrictive drawdown, while other grantees with fewer site visits had. In fact, two grantees that were placed on restrictive drawdown in 2011 did not have a HRSA site visit at any time from 2008 through 2011.

Third, some of the grantees that HRSA visited most during these 4 years had relatively small grant awards, indicating fewer people being served by that grantee, which suggests that the agency did not prioritize site visits based on grant funding level. For instance, the Virgin Islands received approximately $1 million in 2011 CARE Act Part B funding, based on an estimated 568 living HIV/AIDS cases at the end of 2009, but HRSA conducted six site visits there over 4 years. In contrast, California received the second largest 2011 grant award, approximately $150 million, based on an estimated 117,869 living HIV/AIDS cases at the end of 2009, but HRSA did not conduct any site visits there over the 4 years. See table 1 for the Part A and Part B grantees with the most HRSA site visits and their 2011 grant award and estimated HIV/AIDS cases, and see appendix II for a complete listing of this information for all Part A and Part B grantees. HRSA officials explained that the Virgin Islands had been placed on restrictive drawdown and had a history of severe problems that included both fiscal and administrative issues and problems with service delivery. However, other Part B grantees, with significantly larger grant awards, and a history of problems during the period covered by our review did not receive a HRSA site visit. Furthermore, the District of Columbia, which received approximately

---

[37]We considered a grantee to have a history of problems if it had been placed on restrictive drawdown, had a relevant finding in their annual single audit, or both from 2008 through 2011, based on data HRSA provided. HRSA officials noted that there could be other indications of grantee problems.

$21 million in 2011 CARE Act Part B funding based on an estimated 17,250 living HIV/AIDS cases at the end of 2009, had a history of problems and would require HRSA to spend little in travel funds to conduct site visits, but received only one visit over the 4 years. HRSA officials stated that there is no direct correlation between the amount of grant funding and the size of a grantee's problems. However, because the Part A and Part B grant awards are based on the number of reported living HIV/AIDS cases in each metropolitan area or state, the grantees with larger awards serve more affected people.

Table 1: Part A and Part B Grantees with the Most HRSA Site Visits, 2008-2011

	2011 grant award	Estimated living HIV/AIDS cases[a]	Total number of HRSA site visits, 2008 - 2011
Part A grantees			
Caguas, P.R.[b]	$1.5 million	1,310	6[c]
Detroit, MI	$8.9 million	9,341	3
Memphis, TN	$6.5 million	6,911	3
Middlesex, NJ	$2.5 million	2,831	3
Ponce, P.R.	$1.8 million	1,929	7[c]
San Juan, P.R.	$15 million	11,291	9[c]
Part B grantees			
Pennsylvania	$43 million	33,661	3
Puerto Rico	$31 million	18,172	10[c]
Virgin Islands	$1.2 million	568	6

Source: GAO analysis of HRSA data

Note: For Part A, 2011 grant awards ranged from approximately $1.8 million to $121 million. For Part B, 2011 grant awards ranged from the statutory minimum of $50,000 for U.S. territories other than Guam and the Virgin Islands to $162 million. See app. II for the number of HRSA site visits for all Part A and B grantees.

[a]Estimated living HIV/AIDS cases as of December 31, 2009. These case counts were used to calculate the 2011 grant award.

[b]Caguas, Puerto Rico lost its classification as a TGA before the 2011 grant year, so the award amount listed is from grant year 2010, the estimated living HIV/AIDS cases are as of December 31, 2008, and the total number of site visits are from 2008 through grant year 2010.

[c]HRSA officials explained that when HRSA staff made trips to Puerto Rico, they generally tried to include stops at one or multiple Part A grantees and/or the Part B grantee. For example, a March 2009 trip to Puerto Rico included a site visit to the Part B grantee, to the San Juan Part A grantee, and to the Caguas Part A grantee. From 2008 through 2011, HRSA made 12 separate trips to Puerto Rico.

Furthermore, HRSA often was not timely in providing site visit follow-up to grantees. HHS guidance states that agencies are to document in writing site visit reports to grantees as soon as possible after completion of the visit. At the time of our file review, HRSA did not have guidance for POs specifying time frames with which to provide site visit reports. Our file review for grant years 2010 and 2011 found that 12 of the PO files for the 13 grantees that received site visits that occurred during that time period contained a copy of the site visit report. However, many of the grantees we interviewed that had a HRSA site visit during the period of our review said that it took HRSA a long time to provide the site visit report. Specifically, 15 of the 25 grantees we interviewed told us they had a HRSA site visit from 2008 through 2011. Eight of those 15 grantees said that it took over 30 days to receive the site visit report; it took HRSA 4 months or longer to provide 6 of those grantees with the site visit report. In a December 2011 update to its Operations Manual, which was not in place during the majority of the period covered by our review, HRSA specified that POs are to provide site visit reports to grantees within 30 days of the visit.

POs Did Not Always Review Annual Single Audit Findings

Some POs we interviewed said that they were not always aware of grantees' single audit findings or corrective actions developed in response to audit findings. According to HHS guidance, HRSA is to review annual single audit reports as part of its grantee oversight, and may use annual single audit information in decisions about implementing special award conditions such as restrictive drawdowns. Though DFI is the HRSA division primarily responsible for helping to ensure that grantees take appropriate corrective actions in response to single audit findings, POs, within HAB, are responsible for providing overall monitoring of grantees' compliance with program requirements. We have found in past work that audits may provide important information on grantee performance and can serve as an accountability mechanism to help determine whether grantees used funds in accordance with program rules and regulations.[38] For this reason, PO monitoring could be enhanced by the timely review of single audit findings.

However, some POs told us that DFI does not consistently share information about single audit findings and corrective actions. Though POs are able to access a summary of a grantee's HRSA-related single audit findings in EHB, the EHB summary does not specify whether the findings are related to CARE Act programs in particular, which might make it difficult for POs to determine whether the audit contains

---

[38]GAO, *Single audit: Survey of CFO Act Agencies*, GAO-02-376 (Washington, D.C.: March 2002).

information pertinent to their monitoring efforts without explanation from DFI. DFI officials told us they may contact POs or other HRSA staff to help review and ensure the adequacy of grantee corrective actions, but according to POs they do not always do so. Given their knowledge of grantees through routine monitoring activities, POs could provide DFI with valuable input regarding grantees' corrective actions. However, one PO told us that DFI did not notify her when the grantees in her portfolio had audit findings, and another told us that DFI did not consistently share grantee corrective action plans in response to audit findings with her, though DFI might on occasion alert her if there was an issue with a grantee audit. One PO reported that she was recently consulted by DFI to provide input into a grantee's audit findings, but added that this was the first time such consultation had occurred. HRSA officials said that they have enhanced the ways in which DFI communicates audit information to POs through EHB by including citations about audit findings specific to CARE Act programs along with grantee corrective actions designed to address the findings. HRSA officials said that they began doing this as of April 30, 2012.

The lack of consistent communication about single audit findings across HRSA divisions limits opportunities for POs to incorporate single audit information into their monitoring and help HRSA ensure that grantees take timely and effective corrective actions, as required. This is especially important given that HRSA may on occasion use single audit findings as a basis for implementing restrictive drawdowns, which require POs to work with grantees in reviewing financial information as part of grantees' drawdown requests, even if the restrictive drawdown was recommended by DFI. In addition, opportunities for POs to help grantees implement timely corrective actions may also be affected by the lengthy time frames of the single audit process. For example, DFI officials told us that a grantee may be cited for a repeat finding in an audit before they have had time to correct the finding from the prior year's audit. We previously reported that in the Single Audit process it could take 15 months or more from the end of the fiscal year in which an audit finding is initially identified before a grantee's corrective action plan is approved by the responsible federal agency.[39] Thus, in some cases, grantees may not have the opportunity to correct audit findings and POs may not have the

---

[39]GAO, *Federal Grants: Improvements Needed in Oversight and Accountability Processes*, GAO-11-773T (Washington, D.C.: June 2011).

opportunity to help ensure that the grantee corrects audit findings before the following year's audit is conducted.

Though single audits may contain information important to PO monitoring of grantees such as an assessment of how grantees are monitoring their service providers or whether the grantee is properly documenting client eligibility, some grantees told us that neither POs nor other HRSA staff generally communicate with them about single audits. Six grantees said that they did not recollect having any communication with HRSA about audit findings, though five others noted they had discussed audit findings with HRSA staff on at least one occasion, including one who said they discussed their annual single audit with HRSA staff during a site visit. Three POs told us that grantees sometimes initiate communication about their single audits. For example, one PO said that although she generally does not get involved with the audits or receive information from DFI, she had been contacted by one of her grantees regarding an audit finding, and therefore reviewed the proposed corrective actions as part of her routine monitoring.

HRSA Did Not Clearly Communicate with Grantees about the Restrictive Drawdown Process

HRSA often did not communicate or document the reasons for implementing a restrictive drawdown. Only 2 of the 11 grantees from our sample of 25 that were on restrictive drawdown said that HRSA communicated the reasons they were placed on restrictive drawdown. In five cases, the grantee said they only learned about the restrictive drawdown upon receiving a new NOA, without prior warning or explanation from their PO or other HRSA staff. Though the issuance of a new NOA is the official means of notifying the grantee of the new condition on their grant award, NOAs do not enumerate the reasons for the restrictive drawdown. Though HRSA officials stated that grantees were notified verbally or in some cases by e-mail about their restrictive drawdown status, we found that the PO files for many of the 11 grantees in our sample that were on restrictive drawdown did not contain documentation of the reasons the restrictive drawdown was imposed. Federal regulations state that when an agency implements a condition on a grantee award such as a restrictive drawdown, it is to notify the grantee of the nature of the condition and the reason it is being imposed, and HHS guidance states that the agency is to document the reasons for use of the condition in the grant file.[40] According to HRSA, 6 of the 52 Part A grantees and 13 of the 59 Part B grantees were on restrictive drawdown from 2008 through 2011.[41]

HRSA also has not consistently provided grantees placed on restrictive drawdown with instructions about how to meet the conditions for drawing down funds. HHS guidance states that the agency is to explain the nature of, and requirements for meeting, the conditions of the restrictive drawdown. However, 5 of the 11 sampled grantees that were on restrictive drawdown told us that HRSA did not provide clear instructions at the time the restriction was imposed for submitting drawdown requests or the supporting documentation they were required to submit with each request. Four grantees said that when they were first put on restrictive drawdown, they had to repeatedly submit their drawdown requests to their PO before clear expectations were established. One grantee said that they believed that HRSA was "making up the rules about restrictive drawdown as they went along," and another stated that they received no guidance or written instruction specifying the documentation required as part of a drawdown request, which caused delays in the processing of their requests.

Further, HRSA has not consistently provided grantees with guidance on the types of corrective actions needed, including time frames for making the required changes, in order to have the restrictive drawdown removed. Federal regulations state that needed corrective actions and timelines are to be explained to the grantee at the time a restrictive drawdown is implemented. Most of the grantees in our sample said that they were not given a written set of action steps or specific corrective actions needed in

---

[40]Federal regulations also specify that when the agency awarding a federal grant imposes conditions on a grantee award such as restrictive drawdowns, the agency will notify the grantee in writing of the nature of the condition, the reasons for imposing it, the required corrective actions and time frames for completing them, and the method for requesting reconsideration of the conditions. HRSA's recently issued guidance, though not in effect during the period of our review, also states that POs are to document their reasons for recommending that a grantee be placed on restrictive drawdown.

[41]Though HRSA has reported that, in accordance with HHS guidance, the GMO/GMS and PO work together in monitoring grantees through activities including reviews of grantee reports and drawdown requests related to restrictive drawdowns, most of the grantees we interviewed told us that they had minimal interaction with their GMS. Though GMO/GMSs and POs may work together to resolve grantee issues within HRSA, HRSA told us that POs are the HRSA staff with the most direct interaction with grantees.

order to have the restrictive drawdown removed. For example, one grantee told us that although they are willing to do what is needed to have the restriction removed, HRSA has not provided them with a set of requirements and timelines either verbally or in writing. Another grantee said that HRSA did not offer training to the grantee on the requirements for its restrictive drawdown until over a year after the condition was imposed. A third grantee stated that though after the restrictive drawdown process they made a change that will help them hold their service providers more accountable, the process would have been more beneficial had they been given a clear picture of the end goals at the outset.

HRSA officials said that when a restrictive drawdown is lifted, the grantee is to be notified through a new NOA which is signed by the GMO. HRSA's recently issued guidance states that the agency will revisit a grantee's restrictive drawdown status once the grantee completes steps such as submitting documentation of compliance with corrective actions, completing recommended TA, and implementing a corrective action plan developed as part of a site visit. However, HRSA has lifted the restrictive drawdown condition for only two of the grantees in our sample since this guidance was in place, and it is unclear whether HRSA provided grantees with a clear plan for the removal of the condition even upon completion of recommended TA or corrective actions. One grantee explained that each time they made the changes requested by HRSA, they were given a new set of requirements to meet. For example, according to a TA report by HRSA consultants about 1 month after the restrictive drawdown was implemented, the grantee had taken important steps to address its financial challenges. Further, documents provided by the grantee indicate that following the consultant TA report, the PO indicated he would recommend that the grantee be removed from restrictive drawdown. However, despite documenting its ongoing work to address its financial challenges, the grantee was told more than a month later that further steps would be required before the condition would be removed, and the grantee remained on restrictive drawdown for approximately 4 more months. The grantee stated that they were not clearly told what they could do to have the condition removed despite repeated requests for that information, and that the costs to the program of remaining on restrictive drawdown interfered with the possible benefits.

HRSA officials said that HRSA is revising the restrictive drawdown language to be included in the NOA to include the reasons for the restriction, needed corrective actions, and the type of documentation required for the drawdown requests to be processed, and would begin using this updated language on NOAs for grantees placed on restrictive drawdown after May 1, 2012. HRSA officials said that grantees are to be informed in writing of all conditions on their awards and how to proceed in order to have the conditions removed. They said that, where that is not occurring, they will work to ensure that it does.

We found that HRSA did not always provide grantees with additional TA or time to correct deficiencies before placing them on restrictive drawdown. HHS guidance states that an agency will generally afford the grantee an opportunity to correct any deficiencies before imposing conditions such as restrictive drawdown. Two grantees told us they were placed on restrictive drawdown after a site visit, but one noted that they were not given an opportunity to address the site visit findings before being placed on restrictive drawdown. The grantee stated that they submitted a corrective action plan in response to site visit findings approximately 2 months after receiving the site visit report, but according to HRSA the grantee was placed on restrictive drawdown right after the plan was submitted, suggesting the grantee did not have an opportunity to implement the corrective action plan before the condition was put in place.

HRSA has stated that the restrictive drawdown process is a means of doing more intensive monitoring of grantees experiencing problems with program implementation, financial management, or other administrative issues. Two of the grantees in our sample told us that they had more frequent communication with their PO during monitoring calls or through e-mails after restrictive drawdown was implemented. In some cases, however, the restrictive drawdown process may have exacerbated a grantee's existing challenges. For example, one grantee said they were told that they were put on restrictive drawdown because they had an unobligated balance that resulted from not spending funds at a quick enough pace. However, the grantee told us that, in part due to a lack of clear instructions from HRSA, the restrictive drawdown process caused further delays in their ability to spend grant funds and therefore aggravated the unobligated balance problem. In another case, a HRSA financial TA consultant reported that the restrictive drawdown itself was causing delays in a grantee's ability to spend its grant funds, which the consultant feared might lead to a finding in the grantee's next single audit.

HRSA's Lack of Records and Changes in PO Assignments Further Challenge Its Oversight of CARE Act Grantees

HRSA's lack of records and frequent staff changes in PO assignments further challenge the agency's oversight of grantees. HRSA officials told us that records of grantee oversight are located across three types of the agency's files— HRSA's EHB, which includes official NOAs and required reports, annual single audit reports, and PO files, which include monitoring documentation, such as notes from routine calls and TA, and site visit reports—not just those documents available electronically in HRSA's EHB. Therefore, we consider all three of these files together to be a complete record of grantee oversight. While conducting our file review, we found that this complete oversight record was only maintained for the current and previous grant years because, prior to that, consistent with its records management program, HRSA destroyed documentation of grantee monitoring only available in the paper PO files. At the time of our file review midway through the 2011 grant year, all three grantee files were only available for the first half of grant year 2011 and grant year 2010, which was only approximately a year and a half of documentation. Therefore, HRSA's ability to correct previously noted problems with grantee performance could be limited because easily accessible documentation of such problems was not maintained. In fact, a HRSA official told us that he believed that one grantee with a history of problems should be placed on restrictive drawdown. However, HRSA did not take this step because they had destroyed the site visit reports containing findings that would have supported placement on restrictive drawdown. In a December 2011 update to HRSA's Operations Manual, which was not in place during the majority of our review, HRSA specified that POs are to maintain copies of site visit reports for at least 5 years, and any documents related to issues under investigation for as long as necessary. However, this change does not apply to other key documentation in PO files, such as regularly scheduled conference calls and copies of relevant emails.

Furthermore, frequent PO changes in monitoring assignments could compound the challenges created by HRSA's lack of long-standing documentation and possibly limit HRSA's institutional memory for a given grantee. Specifically, according to HRSA data, from 2008 through 2011,

93 of the 111 Part A and Part B grantees had at least two or three different POs and 2 grantees had four different POs during this time.[42]

HRSA's frequent changes in PO assignments could leave a recently transitioned PO and his new grantee at a disadvantage. For example, during our file review, we found that one of the grantees in our sample, a grantee with a history of problems that had been placed on restrictive drawdown, was missing documentation of monitoring calls for the 2010 grant year. That grantee's current PO began monitoring the grantee near the beginning of the 2011 grant year and she explained that she did not receive documentation of any monitoring calls that had occurred under the previous PO.

Some of the grantees we interviewed said that frequent PO changes resulted in variation in HRSA oversight. Eight of the 25 grantees we spoke with expressed concern about changes in their POs and 13 described the variation in PO monitoring styles that grantees had to adjust to when a new PO was assigned. For example, 1 grantee that had three POs from 2008 through 2011 told us that the PO changes resulted in delayed responses from HRSA and contradictory information being provided by different POs, which created confusion for the grantee and delays in funding distribution to service providers. Conversely, a grantee that had one PO during this time period told us that having a knowledgeable PO who serves for a long period of time creates better management of the grant because the PO develops important institutional memory about the grantee and its program.

---

[42]Four Part A grantees lost their classification as TGAs before the 2011 grant year. Of these four grantees, one had a single PO from 2008 through 2011, two had two POs during this time period, and one had three POs during this time period.

HRSA Recently Issued National Standards for Grantee Monitoring of Service Providers, but HRSA's Implementation Created Challenges for Grantees

Federal regulations require grantees to oversee service providers and, in April 2011, HRSA issued the National Monitoring Standards, a compilation of requirements for grantee monitoring of service providers. Some grantees said that their implementation of the standards was hindered by insufficient HRSA assistance and the annual site visit requirement.

Grantees Monitor Service Providers and HRSA Recently Issued National Standards

Federal regulations require grantees to oversee service providers. HRSA told us that grantees are required to report to HRSA on their approach to service provider monitoring activities in annual grant applications. HRSA also verifies this information through grantee site visits and a review of a list of service providers, which grantees are required to submit annually.[43] The number of service providers for Part A and Part B grantees ranges greatly. For example, Nebraska had only 3 service providers in 2011, whereas New York had 83 providers. Grantees we interviewed said they use a variety of tools to monitor their service providers, including frequent phone and e-mail communication, monthly service provider meetings, site visits, training, or reviews of financial and program reports. Specifically, most of the 25 grantees we interviewed told us that they are in at least monthly, if not daily, communication with their service providers. In addition, all but four grantees conduct service provider site visits at least annually. Of the four grantees that were not conducting site visits annually, two large states conducted site visits every 2 years, with one of those states visiting service providers with performance issues more frequently; one midsize state conducted site visits every 3 years; and one small state had not conducted site visits in many years. However, all but one of these grantees were in the process of beginning annual site visits at the time of our interview.

In April 2011, HRSA issued the National Monitoring Standards, which it describes as a compilation of existing requirements for grantee monitoring of Part A and Part B service providers. The standards include

---

[43]This list of service providers is called the Consolidated List of Contractors. For a description of this reporting requirement, see app. I.

133 requirements for Part A grantees and 154 requirements for Part B grantees. These standards describe program and financial requirements, program-only requirements, and financial-only requirements. (See table 2.)

Table 2: Summary of HRSA's National Monitoring Standards for Grantee Monitoring of Service Providers

Type of National Monitoring Standard	Number of Part A standards	Number of Part B standards
Program and financial monitoring standards	19	19
Program-only monitoring standards	51	65
Financial-only monitoring standards	63	70
Total	**133**	**154**

Source: HRSA

According to HRSA, these standards consist of preexisting requirements for program and financial management, monitoring, and reporting that are based on federal statutes, regulations, and program guidance and consolidates these requirements into one location to assist grantees. Table 3 provides examples of the standards.

Table 3: Examples of HRSA's National Monitoring Standards and Grantee Responsibilities for Part A and Part B Grantee Monitoring of Service Providers, by Topic

National Monitoring Standards topic	Example of a standard from selected topics[a]	Examples of grantee responsibilities to ensure service provider compliance with the standard
Examples of program and financial monitoring standards		
Access to care	Grantee must ensure that services are provided by the service provider regardless of the current or past health condition of clients.	• Review provider eligibility policies. • Investigate any relevant provider complaints.
Eligibility	Grantee must ensure that service providers screen and reassess client eligibility as specified by the EMA, TGA, state, or ADAP every 6 months.	• Establish an EMA, TGA, or statewide process for determining client eligibility. • Conduct service provider site visits to review client files for appropriate documentation of eligibility.
Monitoring	Grantee service provider monitoring activities are expected to include annual site visits.	• Use a combination of program reports, annual site visits, client satisfaction reviews, technical assistance, and chart reviews to monitor service provider program compliance.
Examples of program-only monitoring standards		
Core medical services	Grantee must ensure that oral health services include diagnostic, preventive, and therapeutic dental care that is in compliance with dental practice laws, includes evidence-based clinical decisions, is based on an oral health treatment plan, adheres to specified service caps, and is provided by licensed and certified dental professionals.	• Develop a request for proposal and contract for the provision of oral health that specifies program requirements, including that services cover diagnostic, preventive, and therapeutic oral health services. • Review client charts for compliance with contract and program requirements.
Support services	Grantee must ensure that health education and risk reduction services are provided to educate clients living with HIV about HIV transmission and how to reduce the risk of HIV transmission.	• Develop a request for proposal and contract that defines risk reduction counseling. • Review provider data to determine compliance with contract.
Other service requirements	Grantee must ensure that service providers set aside specific amounts for care of women, infants, children, and youth based on the population's relative percentage of the total number of persons living with AIDS in the EMA, TGA, or state.[b]	• Track and report the amount and percentage of CARE Act funds expended for each population group separately.
Examples of financial-only monitoring standards		
Limitations on uses of funding	Grantee must ensure that service providers assign appropriate expenses as administrative expenses, such as usual and recognized overhead activities (rent, utilities, and facility costs).[c]	• Maintain file documentation on all service providers, including current operating budgets and allocation reports that include sufficient detail to identify and calculate administrative expenses. • Review service provider expense reports to ensure that all administrative costs are allowable.

National Monitoring Standards topic	Example of a standard from selected topics[a]	Examples of grantee responsibilities to ensure service provider compliance with the standard
Income from fees for services performed	Grantee must ensure that service providers are using third party funds, such as Medicaid, the Children's Health Insurance Program, Medicare, and private insurance, to maximize program income and ensure that Ryan White is the payer of last resort.	• Establish and implement a process to ensure that service providers maximize third party reimbursements by, for example, requiring service providers to document in client files how each client was screened for and enrolled in eligible insurance programs.
Imposition and assessment of client charges	Grantee must ensure that no charges are imposed on clients with incomes below 100 percent of the Federal Poverty Level.[d]	• Review service provider discount fee policy, criteria, and forms. • Review client files and documentation of actual charges and payments.

Source: HRSA

[a]This table lists examples of HRSA's National Monitoring Standards and is not an exhaustive list of each standard.

[b]A women, infants and children waiver is available if the grantee can document that funds sufficient to meet the needs of these population groups are being provided through other federal or state programs.

[c]Grantees must ensure that service providers adhere to the requirement that aggregated administrative expenses do not total more than 10 percent of CARE Act service dollars.

[d]Federal poverty level refers to the federal poverty guidelines which are used to establish eligibility for certain federal assistance programs. HHS publishes these guidelines on an annual basis, updating the guidelines to reflect changes in the cost of living and variations according to family size.

Implementation of Monitoring Standards Hindered by Insufficient Assistance from HRSA and Challenged by the Annual Site Visit Requirement

More than half of the 25 grantees from our sample said that they found the training and/or TA HRSA has provided on the National Monitoring Standards to be insufficient because it has not answered all of their questions about HRSA's expectations for how they should implement the standards. According to HRSA officials, HRSA has offered two webinars, a national TA call, and workshops at an all-grantees meeting to assist grantees. Some grantees told us HRSA also discussed the standards during a recent administrative meeting. Further, 5 of the 10 POs we interviewed told us they had discussed implementation of the standards with grantees during routine monitoring. Five grantees told us they had asked for more in-depth TA on the standards but had not received it. One grantee, however, did receive additional TA by phone from a HRSA branch chief targeted to all Part A and Part B providers in the grantee's state. Although HRSA stated that it would provide sample tools to demonstrate how grantees could best meet certain standards, several grantees indicated that HRSA had not done so. According to most grantees, inadequate training, TA, or both makes it more difficult to understand HRSA's expectations and be assured that they are adequately implementing the standards, which they were required to put into practice immediately upon their release in April 2011. HRSA officials said that they believe that the webinars, conference call, and presentations they have made at grantee meetings have provided grantees with useful assistance in implementing the standards. They further noted that the standards do not represent new requirements and therefore should have been familiar to grantees. However, in its survey of grantees, discussed earlier in this report, HRSA asked grantees about their training needs and any additional information needs they might have regarding a variety of issues, including the standards.

Seven grantees expressed particular concern about the annual site visit requirement outlined in the standards, which two of them noted is especially challenging for grantees with a large number of providers across a large geographic area or in states with limited staff resources. Two of those grantees said that the new standard would require them to change site visit processes that had proven effective over time. They told us that they conduct routine site visits based on an assessment of risk; if they determine through regular monitoring that a provider has more performance issues than other providers, they will prioritize a site visit to that provider or visit that provider more frequently. They said that the requirement to visit every service provider annually, regardless of their performance, will not allow them to continue with this approach. One grantee with approximately 140 service providers told us that meeting the annual site visit requirement would be impossible given the grantee's large number of providers and limited staff and administrative resources. One grantee told us the administrative burden of this requirement is exacerbated by the chart review requirements which will require grantees to spend more time reviewing provider documents on site, while sacrificing other monitoring activities focused on the quality of provider services. Two grantees noted that the annual site visit standard is more stringent than HRSA's own standard for site visits to grantees, and that HRSA therefore may not have a good sense of the time and resources required to conduct annual site visits of all service providers. Despite these concerns, several grantees told us they are taking steps to comply with the requirement.

NASTAD has written that the standards will require some grantees to largely restructure current monitoring systems and force them to focus on administrative reviews rather than an assessment of the quality of services being delivered by service providers, and that the standards are inconsistent with the National HIV/AIDS Strategy's goal of streamlining grant administration and reporting requirements.[44] NASTAD has further noted that the annual site visit requirement will be especially difficult for grantees during a time when grantees are experiencing reductions in funding and staff, and that the requirement will force grantees to dedicate limited staff resources toward monitoring activities rather than service delivery. According to NASTAD, grantees may also find it difficult to conduct all required provider monitoring activities using only the 10 percent of their CARE Act grant allowed for administrative costs.[45] Many grantees also told us that the standards increase the administrative burden on their programs. HRSA responded to NASTAD that grantees should review their current use of administrative resources to ensure they are efficiently using resources to meet all of the monitoring standards, which are simply meant to provide clarity about existing requirements. In light of grantees' ongoing concerns, however, NASTAD has recommended that HRSA explore alternatives to the annual site visit requirement, including requiring a site visit every 2 years instead of annually. In response to NASTAD's recommendations, HRSA has stated that annual provider site visits are a programmatic requirement developed based on federal regulations permitting HRSA to set the frequency of monitoring activities, including site visits. HRSA also stated that the site visit requirement, which is consistent for all Part A and Part B grantees, is based on HHS OIG recommendations that HRSA set standards for grantee monitoring of service providers that include some consideration of regular site visits.[46] NASTAD has written that because HRSA has

[44]The National HIV/AIDS strategy is a national plan for reducing new HIV infections, improving access to care and health outcomes for people living with HIV, and reducing HIV-related health disparities. It is coordinated by the White House Office of National AIDS Policy. The July 2010 National HIV/AIDS Strategy Federal Implementation Plan outlines key steps for achieving strategic goals, including increasing coordination of HIV program across the federal government and between federal agencies and state, territorial, local, and tribal governments.

[45]The CARE Act requires that grantees spend no more than 10 percent of their grant on administrative activities, which include TA and service provider monitoring activities. 42 U.S.C. §§ 300ff-14(h), 300ff-28(b)(3). The cost of conducting service provider site visits must therefore be included in that 10 percent of the grant.

[46]U.S. Department of Health and Human Services. Office of Inspector General. "Monitoring of Ryan White CARE Act Title I & Title II Grantees" (Washington, D.C.: U.S. Government Printing Office, 2004). http://oig.hhs.gov/oei/reports/oei-02-01-00640.pdf and U.S. Department of Health and Human Services. Office of Inspector General. "The Ryan White CARE Act Title I and Title II Grantees' Monitoring of of Subgrantees" (Washington, D.C.: U.S. Government Printing Office, 2004). http://oig.hhs.gov/oei/reports/oei-02-01-00641.pdf

authority to set the frequency of monitoring activities, it should consider alternatives to the annual site visit requirement.

In response to grantee concerns about the standards, HRSA officials have stated that TA may be requested through individual POs, and that it will provide future webinars focused on common grantee concerns, including the annual site visit requirement and eligibility documentation. HRSA officials further told us that they are encouraging collaboration between Part A and Part B grantees to jointly conduct site visits of providers that are funded by both Parts A and B to ease the burden of the site visit requirement. At least one larger grantee told us they will take advantage of that opportunity for collaboration. Some grantees stated that the standards are a helpful tool, and a few noted that the standards will help them better communicate with their service providers.

Conclusions

Effective oversight of CARE Act grantees and service providers is critical to the CARE Act's mission of providing help for uninsured or underinsured individuals and families affected by HIV/AIDS. However, our findings show that deficiencies in HRSA's oversight may compromise its ability to ensure that this program is meeting its objectives or that CARE Act funds are being spent properly. Even though HHS and HRSA guidance exists regarding the documentation and follow-up of the key elements of grantee oversight including routine monitoring, the provision of TA, site visits, and restrictive drawdown, HRSA project officers are not always following these guidelines. If a grantee is struggling, the lack of systematic provision and documentation of assistance to improve the grantee's performance, and not retaining such documentation over time, present a great challenge to ensuring that such problems do not recur. Many HRSA POs we spoke with said that site visits are a valuable and effective oversight tool. However, in visiting some grantees multiple times while not visiting others, seemingly without regard to the size of the grantee or presence of problems, HRSA demonstrated a lack of a strategic, risk-based approach for selecting grantees for site visits. Another challenge is the lack of an updated and electronically available comprehensive program manual for grantees. Grantees said that such a manual would likely decrease their need to consult with POs over relatively routine issues. Currently, grantees must frequently seek assistance from POs because there is not a current and complete source of written information that is readily available to guide their efforts. While HRSA's compilation of 133 Part A and 154 Part B monitoring standards does provide grantees with an exhaustive set of guidelines for ensuring that their service providers are meeting program requirements, our findings on HRSA's own oversight of grantees provide evidence of how important training and follow-up are to ensure that these requirements are consistently followed. HRSA has provided training to assist grantees in carrying out the standards, but grantees said that they wanted more guidance and training. Among the issues about which HRSA surveyed its grantees, was the additional information its grantees needed regarding the standards.

Recommendations for Executive Action

In order to improve HRSA's oversight of Part A and Part B grantees, we recommend that the Administrator of HRSA:

- Ensure that the agency is implementing the key elements of grantee oversight consistent with HHS and HRSA guidance, including routine monitoring, the provision of technical assistance, site visits, and restrictive drawdown.

- Assess and revise its record retention management program so that complete grantee files are available for a period of time that HRSA determines will satisfy all of the agency's grantee oversight needs.

- Develop a strategic, risk-based approach for selecting grantees for site visits that better targets the use of available resources to ensure that HRSA visits grantees at regular and timely intervals.

- Update and maintain a program manual for grantees.

- Use the results of HRSA's survey of grantees to identify grantees' training needs to allow them to comply with the National Monitoring Standards.

Agency Comments and Our Evaluation

We provided a draft of this report to HHS for its review, and HHS provided written comments (see app III). HHS concurred with all five of our recommendations and indicated that HRSA will work to fully implement the recommendations to improve oversight of Parts A and B of the CARE Act program. HHS also offered some specific comments in response to the report conclusions. HHS acknowledged that PO led site visits, monitoring calls, single audit reports, and the imposition of restrictive drawdown are central to HRSA's routine monitoring, but added that the agency's overall oversight strategy is a multilayered approach that involves review of items such as required grantee reports used for postaward monitoring, site visits, monitoring calls, review of audit reports, and the provision of technical assistance on all of these issues. Our analysis included these elements, as well as a discussion of ways in which these elements intersect. We interviewed HRSA and grantee staff on these tools and describe in this report grantees' observations on HRSA's provision of technical assistance and feedback on the large number of reports that they must routinely provide to HRSA. Findings in this report include a detailed discussion of issues in Ryan White program oversight including both the execution and documentation of the elements listed above.

HHS also acknowledged that HRSA's documentation of grantee monitoring should be strengthened, noting that during the period of GAO's review, HRSA did not maintain all documentation of oversight in one centralized file. HHS stated that HRSA has instituted a new quality improvement process, which strengthens both documentation standards and communication with grantees. HHS said that this would be done through an expansion of the use of the EHB as the primary centralized location for documentation of oversight and monitoring, including site visit reports. HHS said that this process will also include regular PO meetings to provide training, and improvements in HRSA's records management practices. These steps appear to be consistent with the goals of our recommendations. In follow-up to its comments, HRSA provided additional information on the agency's planned information technology development efforts to improve and expand the functionality of EHB between September 2012 and mid-2013.

HHS commented on statements by grantees we interviewed that indicated that HRSA could not provide needed TA due to budget constraints, forcing the four grantees to seek TA from other sources, using their own administrative funds. HHS described a wide array of TA and training services that HRSA provides to grantees. HHS also provided information on the extent of grantees' use of some of these services and HRSA's financial resources devoted to providing these services. HHS acknowledged in this discussion that, due to competing demands for HRSA's TA, HRSA does, at times, recommend grantees utilize their CARE Act funding for TA. In its comments relevant to TA, HHS also noted our mention of the fact that three grantees had to turn to NASTAD for TA when HRSA could not provide it or when PO responses to their questions were delayed. HHS noted that HRSA has had a partnership with NASTAD in place since 1998 to provide TA to grantees. However, as we note in our report, the TA to be provided by NASTAD under this partnership is for the purpose of assisting Part B grantees with their ADAP. While several Part B grantees told us that they receive important assistance from NASTAD, there is no similar cooperative agreement in place or HRSA-recognized organization to provide TA to Part A grantees.

HHS also commented on our finding that HRSA did not prioritize site visits strategically. HHS stated that there can be indications of grantee problems beyond those that we included in our site visit analysis, which we acknowledged in the report. Many of the additional indicators of grantee problems HHS listed in its comments, such as fiscal and administrative challenges, are also issues that can cause grantees to receive annual single audit findings or to be placed on restrictive drawdown, the two indicators we used in our analysis. HHS then provided extensive detail on the issues in Puerto Rico and the Virgin Islands that led to grantees in those jurisdictions receiving significantly more site visits than other grantees that had received substantially more funding. In our discussion of HRSA's site visits, we make the point that the size of the grant did not appear to play a major role in HRSA's decisions about which grantees to visit, including among grantees experiencing problems. Many POs we spoke with said that site visits were a valuable and effective form of oversight. Because HRSA cannot visit all of its grantees each year, it must work to ensure that it uses this valuable tool in such a way as to gain as much benefit as possible. The Monitoring Grants and Cooperative Agreements for Federal Personnel manual that we refer to in the report and HHS cites in its comments lists several grant characteristics that should be considered in selecting projects for on-site monitoring. "Cost and Total Support" is the first issue listed in the manual. In our discussion, we did not question the presence of serious issues in Puerto Rico and the Virgin Islands. Our point is that even among grantees experiencing problems, jurisdictions with much larger grants, such as the District of Columbia, were not similarly prioritized for site visits, even though a site visit to the District of Columbia would be of low cost to the agency.

HHS commented on the prevalence of HIV/AIDS in the Caribbean as a justification for its numerous site visits, but we note that the size of Part A and B CARE Act grants is based upon the number of HIV cases that exist in the jurisdiction being served by the CARE Act grantee, thereby serving as a proxy for the prevalence of the disease in that area. Data on HRSA's website indicate that CARE Act programs served 146 clients in the Virgin Islands in 2008, while serving 16,203 in the District of Columbia during the same period. HRSA's pattern of site visits indicates that the agency visited some grantees with smaller grants far more often than other grantees with much larger grants, and thus a much higher prevalence of disease, that also experienced challenges in administering their grants. In its comments, HHS describes numerous elements of HRSA's routine monitoring and several instances of TA directed to the District of Columbia. Nonetheless, it received one HRSA site visit during the period covered by our review as compared to the Virgin Islands, which received six HRSA site visits, as well as routine monitoring and TA. The District of Columbia's grant was approximately $21 million while the Virgin Islands' grant was $1.2 million. This suggests that HRSA did not consider the size of the grant in deciding which grantees to visit. While the size of the grant would not be the only consideration in a strategic approach to scheduling site visits, it should be a major consideration.

HHS's comments also addressed the issue of PO's awareness of single audit findings. HHS described how, under HRSA's process during the time covered by our review, POs were to be informed about single audit findings. HHS described an enhancement to HRSA's process for ensuring that POs are provided with a more detailed description of single audit findings and corrective actions taken to address the findings. HHS said that this improved process was put in place as of April 30, 2012, which was after the period covered by our review.

In its comments, HHS also describes improvements to HRSA's documentation of and communication with grantees about the restrictive drawdown process, issues which we already discuss in our report. If fully implemented, these improvements have the potential to remedy many of the issues we identified in our report.

In acknowledging our findings on HRSA's records retention practices, HHS said that HRSA was required to retain records according to schedules approved by the National Archives and Records Administration (NARA). However, it further noted that HRSA has engaged in a review of its records management practices. HHS said that, in December 2011, during the course of our review, HRSA formed a workgroup on records management with program and grant staff across the agency to streamline various retention schedules for program and grant record retention practices. HHS said that HRSA will be providing additional training and updated policies for the HAB POs and grants management specialists on the contents of the official grant file. HHS said that HRSA would seek approval for any changes to HRSA's record retention policies.

In commenting on our discussion of the difficulty some grantees expressed about meeting the requirement for an annual visit of their service providers, HHS noted that HRSA is working with a small number of grantees to provide flexibility in meeting the requirement, but did not describe what that flexibility would entail. In discussions near the end of our review, HRSA officials said that this would not include excusing grantees from the requirement that they visit all of their service providers annually, but could involve leveraging the efforts of other CARE Act grantees.

HHS concluded its general comments on the report by again noting that the department concurred with all five of our recommendations. HHS further commented that HHS is already in the process of planning or implementing many of our recommendations. In its comments, HHS provided considerable detail on actions HRSA plans to take or has already taken to implement our recommendations. The actions HHS describes are generally responsive to our recommendations. However, because these actions follow the conclusion of our review or are to be implemented in the future, and sometimes without a designated time frame, we are unable to evaluate them specifically.

HHS also provided technical comments, which we incorporated as appropriate.

As agreed with your offices, unless you publicly announce the contents of this report earlier, we plan no further distribution until 30 days from the report date. At that time, we will send copies of this report to the Administrator of HRSA and the appropriate congressional committees. In addition, the report is available at no charge on the GAO website at http://www.gao.gov.

If you or your staff have any questions about this report, please contact me at (202) 512-7114 or crossem@gao.gov. Contact points for our Offices of Congressional Relations and Public Affairs may be found on the last page of this report. GAO staff who made major contributions to this report are listed in appendix IV.

Marcia Crosse
Director, Health Care

Appendix I: Reporting Requirements for Part A and Part B Grantees

Table 4: Reporting Requirements for Part A and Part B Grantees, Fiscal Year 2012

Reporting Requirement	Part A	Part B	Date Due for Fiscal Year 2012
AIDS Drug Assistance Program (ADAP) Quarterly Report		✓	July 29, 2011[a]
The ADAP quarterly reports provide aggregate data for ADAP service utilization.		✓	October 31, 2011
		✓	January 31, 2012
		✓	April 30, 2012
Minority AIDS Initiative Annual Plan	✓	✓	Part A: October 17, 2011
The primary Purpose of the Part A MAI Annual Plan is to ensure funds are used to link minority clients to HIV Care services. The primary purpose of the Part B MAI Annual Plan is to ensure funds are used to link minority clients into ADAP services. The plan is to include a planned timeframe for delivering services; a description of service goals and objectives; the racial and ethnic communities to be served and the number of service units to be provided during the reporting period.			Part B: October 7, 2011
Mid-year Progress Report		✓	October 31, 2011
The primary purpose of the mid-year progress report is to inform POs of progress made in administration of the Part B programs; to identify accomplishments and challenges in meeting established goals and objectives; and to address grantees' need for technical assistance.			
Maintenance of Effort Expenditures Report	✓		December 5, 2011
The maintenance of effort expenditures report is used to ensure grantees have maintained level expenditures for two consecutive grant years. The expenditures must be based on the local budget items.			
Program Terms Report	✓	✓	December 5, 2011
The program terms report includes a planned allocation report, budget and budget narrative justification, an implementation plan, the Consolidated List of Contractors and the Contract Review Certification.			
• The allocation report serves as a monitoring tool to track and monitor the use of funds. It identifies categories of services that are being delivered, changes in the type of services being provided over time and trends in the amount of CARE Act funds being used to deliver these services.			
• The budget and budget narrative justification serve as monitoring tools to track and monitor the use of CARE Act funds.			
• The implementation plan serves as a monitoring tool to verify implementation of approved medical and support services for the current grant year. The plan should include all the services and priorities reflected in the allocations report. All funded services must be included in the implementation plan.			
• The Consolidated List of Contractors serves as a list of all funded service providers for the current grant year.			
• The Contract Review Certification requires the grantee to certify that all grant funded service providers for the current grant year comply with CARE Act program requirements, and federal grants requirements.			

Reporting Requirement	Part A	Part B	Date Due for Fiscal Year 2012
Unobligated Balance Estimate and Carryover Request The CARE Act provides that base and supplemental grant funds were available for obligation by the grantee for a 1-year period beginning on the first day of the grant year. It also requires HRSA to cancel any unobligated balances at the end of the grant year, recover funds that had been disbursed to grantees, and redistribute these funds to grantees in need as supplemental grants. Grantees must estimate their unobligated balances during the grant year and provide final amounts in their federal financial report. Grantees may request to carryover funds for one additional grant year.	✓	✓	Part A: January 1, 2012 Part B: January 31, 2012
Interim Federal Financial Report The purpose of the interim financial report is to substantiate that the grantee has obligated 75 percent of the awarded funds for the current grant year.		✓	January 3, 2012
Ryan White HIV/AIDS Program Services Report The Ryan White HIV/AIDS program services report provides information on services provided by grantees and service providers to HRSA. Additionally, grantees and service providers use this report to provide information on clients, including their demographic status, services received and HIV clinical information.	✓	✓	March 15, 2012
Part A Comprehensive Plan The comprehensive plan is a legislative requirement that is due every 3 years at the beginning of the grant year. The plan is to be used as a "road map" for the maintenance and improvement of the grantee's system of care. Grantees are required to include appropriate strategies, goals and timelines.	✓		May 21, 2012
Statewide Coordinated Statement of Need (SCSN) The SCSN is a written statement of need developed through a locally chosen collaborative process with other CARE Act grant parts. The purpose of the SCSN is to provide a collaborative mechanism to identify and address significant HIV care issues related to the needs of people living with HIV/AIDS, and to maximize coordination, integration, and effective linkages across the CARE Act parts. The SCSN process should consider all CARE Act resources within the state, including the amount of funds, as well as the services these funds are support.		✓	June 1, 2012
Final Expenditure Table, including MAI expenditures This expenditure table serves as a monitoring tool to identify the use of funds at the end of the grant period. It identifies service categories that have been delivered, the use of carry-over funds and identifies trends in the amount of CARE Act funds being used to deliver these services.	✓	✓	Part A: June 28, 2012 Part B: September 28, 2012
Federal Financial Report The Federal Financial Report outlines the grantee's outlays, unliquidated obligations, total federal share and final unobligated balance.	✓	✓	Part A: July 30, 2012 Part B: July 30, 2012
Annual Progress Report The Annual Progress Report is to inform POs of the progress made in the administration of Ryan White programs; to identify accomplishments and challenges in meeting established goals and objectives; and to address grantees' need for technical assistance.	✓	✓	Part A: June 28, 2012 Part B: September 28, 2012

Reporting Requirement	Part A	Part B	Date Due for Fiscal Year 2012
Report on Expenditures for Women, Infants, Children and Youth	✓	✓	Part A: July 28, 2012
The report on expenditures for Women, Infants, Children and Youth is a legislative requirement used to determine that a grantee allocates resources for women, infants, children and youth at no less than the percentage constituted by the ratio of the population of women, infants, children and youth with HIV/AIDS to the general populations with HIV/AIDS.			Part B: September 28, 2012
Minority AIDS Initiative Annual Report	✓	✓	Part A: January 31, 2013[b]
Part A and B grantees receiving MAI funds must submit two components of the MAI Report annually: (1) the MAI Annual Plan for the use of these funds, and (2) the year-end MAI Annual Report documenting program outcomes. Each MAI Report has two parts: (1) Web forms for standardized quantitative and qualitative information and (2) an accompanying narrative providing background information to explain the data submitted and a summary of program accomplishments, challenges, and lessons.			Part B: September 28, 2012

Source: HRSA.

Note: The federal 2012 fiscal year was from October 1, 2011, through September 30, 2012. HRSA uses the federal fiscal year to determine when grantee reports are due. However, CARE Act grants have their own grant years. The grant year for Part A is from March 1 through February 28. The Part B grant year is from April 1 through March 31.

[a]The July 29, 2011, AIDS Drug Assistance Program (ADAP) Quarterly Report is due in federal fiscal year 2011.

[b]The Minority AIDS Initiative Annual Report for Part A grantees is due on January 31, 2012, which is in federal fiscal year 2013.

Appendix II: HRSA Site Visits of Part A and Part B Grantees

	2011 Grant award (dollars)	Estimated living HIV/AIDS cases[a]	Number of HRSA site visits, 2008	Number of HRSA site visits, 2009	Number of HRSA site visits, 2010	Number of HRSA site visits, 2011	Total number of HRSA site visits, 2008 – 2011
Atlanta, GA	$21,468,517	22,794	0	0	0	1	1
Austin, TX	4,400,041	4,483	0	0	0	0	0
Baltimore, MD	19,867,958	21,834	1	0	0	1	2
Baton Rouge, LA	3,699,040	4,152	0	0	0	0	0
Bergen-Passaic, NJ	4,044,886	4,296	0	0	1	0	1
Boston, MA	13,769,366	14,992	0	0	0	0	0
Caguas, P.R.[b]	1,524,285	1,310	0	2	3	1	6[c]
Charlotte-Gastonia, NC-SC	5,748,542	5,859	0	0	0	0	0
Chicago, IL	25,986,577	27,451	0	1	1	0	2
Cleveland, OH	3,997,596	4,252	0	0	2	0	2
Dallas, TX	14,570,875	16,288	1	1	0	0	2
Denver, CO	7,826,960	8,452	0	0	0	0	0
Detroit, MI	8,924,079	9,341	1	1	1	0	3
Dutchess County, NY[b]	1,347,313	1,292	0	0	0	1	1
Fort Lauderdale, FL	15,005,889	16,513	0	0	0	0	0
Fort Worth, TX	3,864,078	4,082	0	0	0	0	0
Hartford, CT	4,249,488	3,635	0	0	0	1	1
Houston, TX	19,735,854	20,934	0	0	0	0	0
Indianapolis, IN	3,908,947	4,124	0	1	0	0	1
Jacksonville, FL	5,805,921	5,860	0	0	0	0	0
Jersey City, NJ	5,074,144	5,089	0	0	1	0	1
Kansas City, MO	4,288,671	4,567	0	0	0	0	0
Las Vegas, NV	5,491,345	6,017	0	0	0	0	0
Los Angeles, CA	40,064,159	43,264	1	0	0	0	1
Memphis, TN	6,534,155	6,911	2	1	0	0	3
Miami, FL	25,053,334	25,855	1	0	0	0	1
Middlesex-Somerset-Hunterdon, NJ	2,503,584	2,831	0	3	0	0	3
Minneapolis-St. Paul, MN	5,608,011	5,722	0	0	0	0	0
Nashville, TN	4,677,970	4,765	0	0	1	0	1
Nassau-Suffolk, NY	6,441,136	6,030	0	0	0	0	0
New Haven, CT	6,956,397	6,137	0	0	0	0	0
New Orleans, LA	7,370,711	7,866	0	0	1	0	1

	2011 Grant award (dollars)	Estimated living HIV/AIDS cases[a]	Number of HRSA site visits, 2008	Number of HRSA site visits, 2009	Number of HRSA site visits, 2010	Number of HRSA site visits, 2011	Total number of HRSA site visits, 2008 – 2011
New York, NY	120,859,664	104,932	0	0	0	1	1
Newark, NJ	13,917,826	13,508	0	1	0	0	1
Norfolk, VA	5,986,127	6,179	1	0	0	0	1
Oakland, CA	6,789,146	7,576	0	1	0	0	1
Orange County, CA	5,968,395	6,572	1	0	0	0	1
Orlando, FL	8,313,970	9,791	0	0	1	0	1
Philadelphia, PA	24,102,413	25,047	0	0	0	0	0
Phoenix, AZ	8,257,524	9,073	1	0	0	0	1
Ponce, P.R.	1,842,886	1,929	1	3	3	0	7[c]
Portland, OR	3,742,527	4,210	0	0	1	0	1
Riverside-San Bernardino, CA	7,356,532	8,742	1	0	0	0	1
Sacramento, CA	2,654,867	3,119	1	0	0	0	1
Saint Louis, MO	6,528,396	6,562	0	1	0	0	1
San Antonio, TX	4,413,440	4,657	0	0	0	0	0
San Diego, CA	11,765,451	12,844	0	0	1	0	1
San Francisco, CA	25,608,437	18,463	0	0	0	0	0
San Jose, CA	2,844,809	3,321	0	0	0	0	0
San Juan, P.R.	15,049,530	11,291	3	2	3	1	9[c]
Santa Rosa, CA[b]	1,169,014	1,330	0	1	0	1	2
Seattle, WA	6,870,026	7,373	0	0	0	0	0
Tampa-St. Petersburg, FL	9,370,009	10,367	0	0	0	0	0
Vineland-Millville-Bridgeton, NJ[b]	897,630	852	0	0	0	0	0
Washington, DC	31,006,866	34,715	0	1	0	0	1
West Palm Beach, FL	8,684,130	7,949	0	0	0	0	0

Source: GAO analysis of HRSA data.

[a]Estimated living HIV/AIDS cases as of December 31, 2009. These case counts were used to calculate the 2011 grant award.

[b]Caguas, P.R., Dutchess County, NY, Santa Rosa, CA, and Vineland-Millville-Bridgeton, NJ lost their classification as TGAs before the 2011 grant year, which began March 1, 2011, so the award amount is from grant year 2010 and the estimated living HIV/AIDS cases are as of December 31, 2008.

[c]HRSA officials explained that when HRSA staff made trips to Puerto Rico that included stops at one or multiple Part A grantees and/or the Part B grantee. For example, a March 2009 trip to Puerto Rico included a site visit to the Part B grantee, to the San Juan Part A grantee, and to the Caguas Part A grantee. From 2008 through 2011, HRSA made 12 separate trips to Puerto Rico.

Table 6: HRSA Site Visits of Part B Grantees, 2008-2011

	2011 Grant award (dollars)	Estimated living HIV/AIDS cases[a]	Number of HRSA site visits, 2008	Number of HRSA site visits, 2009	Number of HRSA site visits, 2010	Number of HRSA site visits, 2011	Total number of HRSA site visits, 2008 – 2011
Alabama	$18,809,782	10,941	0	0	0	0	0
Alaska	1,134,180	658	0	0	0	0	0
American Samoa	50,000	2	0	0	0	0	0
Arizona	15,534,483	12,068	0	1	0	0	1
Arkansas	8,373,354	4,992	0	1	0	0	1
California	148,168,287	117,869	0	0	0	0	0
Colorado	14,202,569	10,972	0	0	0	0	0
Connecticut	14,571,752	11,068	0	0	0	0	0
Delaware	5,790,675	3,087	1	0	0	0	1
District of Columbia	21,101,829	17,250	0	1	0	0	1
Federated States of Micronesia	50,000	6	0	0	0	0	0
Florida	126,286,273	97,463	1	0	0	1	2
Georgia	45,331,646	34,733	0	0	0	1	1
Guam	286,530	97	0	0	0	0	0
Hawaii	3,583,940	2,228	0	0	0	0	0
Idaho	1,315,589	780	0	0	0	0	0
Illinois	41,738,721	32,322	0	1	0	0	1
Indiana	11,811,918	8,689	0	1	0	0	1
Iowa	2,933,874	1,759	1	0	0	0	1
Kansas	3,656,596	2,825	0	0	0	0	0
Kentucky	8,304,138	4,777	0	0	0	1	1
Louisiana	23,144,643	17,644	0	0	1	1	2
Maine	1,733,995	1,084	0	0	1	1	2
Marshall Islands	50,000	1	0	0	0	0	0
Maryland	40,187,548	34,379	0	0	0	0	0
Massachusetts	20,457,176	16,929	0	0	0	1	1
Michigan	17,823,185	14,216	0	1	0	0	1
Minnesota	7,711,593	6,488	0	1	0	0	1
Mississippi	12,080,715	8,334	0	0	1	0	1
Missouri	14,157,823	11,584	0	0	0	0	0
Montana	856,281	374	0	1	0	0	1
Northern Mariana Islands	50,000	10	0	0	0	0	0

	2011 Grant award (dollars)	Estimated living HIV/AIDS cases[a]	Number of HRSA site visits, 2008	Number of HRSA site visits, 2009	Number of HRSA site visits, 2010	Number of HRSA site visits, 2011	Total number of HRSA site visits, 2008 – 2011
Nebraska	2,728,244	1,609	0	0	0	0	0
Nevada	8,462,067	7,024	0	0	0	0	0
New Hampshire	1,507,461	1,139	0	0	1	0	1
New Jersey	46,624,149	35,467	0	1	0	0	1
New Mexico	4,019,762	2,487	1	0	0	0	1
New York	162,437,735	130,091	0	1	0	0	1
North Carolina	34,992,574	24,308	0	0	0	0	0
North Dakota	378,141	187	0	0	0	0	0
Ohio	24,817,612	16,997	0	0	0	0	0
Oklahoma	8,431,948	4,840	0	1	0	0	1
Oregon	6,664,158	5,163	0	0	0	0	0
Pennsylvania	43,068,009	33,661	0	3	0	0	3
Puerto Rico	31,376,731	18,172	3	3	2	0	10[b]
Republic of Palau	50,000	3	0	0	0	0	0
Rhode Island	3,962,190	2,555	0	0	2	0	2
South Carolina	25,815,827	14,746	0	0	0	2	2
South Dakota	883,908	403	0	0	0	0	0
Tennessee	20,350,806	15,578	0	0	1	1	2
Texas	85,169,848	66,002	0	0	0	0	0
Utah	3,775,386	2,336	0	0	0	0	0
Vermont	893,492	403	0	0	0	1	1
Virgin Islands	1,161,007	568	1	3	2	0	6
Virginia	27,770,365	20,574	1	0	0	0	1
Washington	13,896,285	10,734	0	0	0	0	0
West Virginia	2,535,511	1,514	0	0	0	0	0
Wisconsin	8,910,774	5,131	0	0	0	0	0
Wyoming	728,630	240	0	0	0	0	0

Source: GAO analysis of HRSA data.

[a]Estimated living HIV/AIDS cases as of December 31, 2009. These case counts were used to calculate the 2011 grant award.

[b]HRSA officials explained that HRSA staff made to Puerto Rico included stops at one or multiple Part A grantees and/or the Part B grantee. For example, a March 2009 trip to Puerto Rico included a site visit to the Part B grantee, to the San Juan Part A grantee, and to the Caguas Part A grantee. From 2008 through 2011, HRSA made 12 separate trips to Puerto Rico.

GAO-12-610 Ryan White CARE Act Oversight

Appendix III: Comments from the Department of Health and Human Services

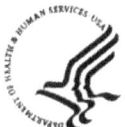
MAY 2 5 2012

Marcia Crosse
Director, Health Care
U.S. Government Accountability Office
441 G Street NW
Washington, DC 20548

Dear Ms. Crosse:

Attached are comments on the U.S. Government Accountability Office's (GAO) report entitled: "RYAN WHITE CARE ACT: Improvements Needed in Oversight of Grantees" (GAO-12-610).

The Department appreciates the opportunity to review this draft section of the report prior to publication.

Sincerely,

Jim R. Esquea
Assistant Secretary for Legislation

Attachment

**GENERAL COMMENTS OF THE DEPARTMENT OF HEALTH AND HUMAN
SERVICES (HHS) ON THE GOVERNMENT ACCOUNTABILITY OFFICE'S
(GAO) DRAFT REPORT ENTITLED, "RYAN WHITE CARE ACT:
IMPROVEMENTS NEEDED IN OVERSIGHT OF GRANTEES" (GAO-12-610)**

Response to the Report's Findings

The Department appreciates the opportunity to review and comment on GAO's draft
report regarding oversight of the Ryan White Human Immunodeficiency Virus/Acquired
Immune Deficiency Syndrome (HIV/AIDS) Program. Administered by the Health
Resources and Services Administration (HRSA), the Ryan White Program provides care,
treatment, and life-saving medications to more than 500,000 men, women, and children
living with HIV/AIDS across the United States. A fuller description of the program is in
Appendix 1.

GAO's report focuses on HRSA's oversight of Part A and Part B of the Ryan White
Program, which by statute provides grants to local and state governments, including the
District of Columbia (D.C.), Puerto Rico, and U.S. Territories. These formula-based
grants support core medical services, including: outpatient and ambulatory medical care;
assistance with paying for life-sustaining medications; oral and behavioral health care;
early intervention services; health insurance assistance; home and community-based
health services; medical case management; and more.

HRSA places great importance on the oversight of grantees. HRSA's program
implementation, and oversight of the program, has resulted in successful outcomes for
people living with HIV/AIDS. The number of clients receiving HIV medical care
through the Ryan White Program has increased nearly 5 percent from 2008-2010.
Among those clients receiving medical care, the Ryan White Program has achieved
significant clinical successes. While many HIV clients struggle to stay on medications,
the proportion of Ryan White Program clients on HIV treatment regimens has increased
from 63 percent in 2008 to 69 percent in 2010. While many people with HIV across the
country are not diagnosed until they have full-blown AIDS, the number of clients in the
Ryan White Program who progressed to AIDS after entering care declined almost 19
percent from 2008 to 2010. Finally, deaths among HIV positive clients receiving Ryan
White Program-funded HIV medical care declined almost 15 percent from 2008 to 2010.

HRSA has a strong commitment to continual and constant review of its own internal
processes and welcomes recommendations from GAO for making the program run more
smoothly and effectively, increasing accountability, and better meeting the health needs
of people living with HIV/AIDS. As a matter of practice, HRSA uses GAO reports on
specific parts of the agency to improve processes agency-wide. In fact, some of the
opportunities for improvement identified by GAO were also identified by HRSA's own

1

**GENERAL COMMENTS OF THE DEPARTMENT OF HEALTH AND HUMAN
SERVICES (HHS) ON THE GOVERNMENT ACCOUNTABILITY OFFICE'S
(GAO) DRAFT REPORT ENTITLED, "RYAN WHITE CARE ACT:
IMPROVEMENTS NEEDED IN OVERSIGHT OF GRANTEES" (GAO-12-610)**

internal review and, as noted in the report, HRSA was already on a course to improve a
number of processes.

Many improvements underway stem from the agency-wide HRSA Program Integrity
Initiative, begun in June 2010, which focuses on identifying and targeting the greatest
risks to grant program performance, reducing those risks through new or enhanced
oversight activities, and identifying and sharing new and best practices. For example, in
2010, HRSA invited the HHS Office of Inspector General (OIG) to conduct a grant fraud
training session attended by over 200 HRSA employees nationwide. As a result, a
comprehensive training program for HRSA's new program integrity analysts was
implemented. Beginning in early FY 2011, HRSA increased program integrity staffing,
both at HRSA's headquarters and in HRSA's ten regional offices, to support the agency
in its monitoring and delivery of financial and technical support to grantees. In addition,
in May of 2011, HRSA hosted a Program Integrity webinar focused on risk and fraud
attended by over 500 grantee participants and over 200 HRSA staff, and partnered with
the Association of Government Accountants on developing a fraud toolkit.

HHS concurs with all five Recommendations for Executive Action and will work to fully
implement those recommendations to improve Ryan White Program oversight. HHS
offers the following specific comments in response to the central conclusions drawn from
the report's findings.

HRSA Does Not Consistently Follow Applicable Guidance for Grantee Oversight.

GAO's review focused on comprehensive, project officer (PO) led site visits, monitoring
calls, single audit reports, and the imposition of restricted draw down. While these
activities are central to HRSA's routine monitoring, HRSA's overall oversight strategy is
a multi-layered approach that involves review of the initial application, required grantee
reports used for post award monitoring, site visits, clinical outcome performance
measures, monitoring calls, review of audit reports, and the provision of technical
assistance on all of these issues. For example, GAO notes that despite a history of
challenges, D.C. only received one comprehensive, PO led site visit during the review
period. However, between 2008 and 2012, D.C. actually received more than ten different
technical assistance visits and/or interventions, including discussions between senior
HRSA officials and the D.C. Commissioner of Health.

2

GENERAL COMMENTS OF THE DEPARTMENT OF HEALTH AND HUMAN SERVICES (HHS) ON THE GOVERNMENT ACCOUNTABILITY OFFICE'S (GAO) DRAFT REPORT ENTITLED, "RYAN WHITE CARE ACT: IMPROVEMENTS NEEDED IN OVERSIGHT OF GRANTEES" (GAO-12-610)

HRSA staff use guidance related to post-award administration and monitoring guidance as set forth in the HHS Awarding Agency Grants Administration Manual. Monitoring guidance specific to HRSA's HIV/AIDS Bureau (HAB) grants is included in the Division of Service Systems (DSS) Operations Manual. The HHS Awarding Agency Grants Administration Manual and the HAB DSS Manual help to ensure integrity and accountability in the award, administration, and oversight of grants. Using these resources, POs, with oversight from their managers, and grants management specialists work together in ongoing monitoring and assessment of Ryan White Program grantees. As described in HRSA's response to GAO's recommendations, the Agency has and will continue to take proactive steps to improve its oversight and monitoring responsibilities.

HRSA Did Not Consistently Document Routine Monitoring.

HHS acknowledges that documentation of grantee monitoring should be strengthened. During the period of GAO's review, HAB did not maintain all documentation of oversight in one centralized file. Three separate grantee files were maintained to assist in the provision of oversight: the PO file, the grant file maintained by the Division of Financial Integrity, and the Electronic Handbook (EHB) – HRSA's electronic grants monitoring system.

During this time, HRSA instituted a new quality improvement process, which strengthens both documentation standards and communication with grantees. As part of the quality improvement process, HAB began expanding the use of the EHB as the primary centralized location for documentation of oversight and monitoring, including site visit reports. This database is accessible to all staff providing oversight to a grant. Moving forward, monitoring activities including review of grantee applications, budgets, progress reports, allocations and expenditures tables, and quarterly reports will be logged centrally in EHB.

The quality improvement process also resulted in instituting bi-monthly PO meetings, where training is provided on topics such as strengthening feedback to grantees on program, fiscal, and service reporting requirements. Lastly, HRSA formed an agency-wide workgroup on records management with program and grant staff across the Agency to review and where needed, strengthen policies and procedures for program and grant record retention practices. HRSA is evaluating best practices across Agency programs in records management policies and procedures and will be using these practices, where needed, in training for project officers.

3

GENERAL COMMENTS OF THE DEPARTMENT OF HEALTH AND HUMAN SERVICES (HHS) ON THE GOVERNMENT ACCOUNTABILITY OFFICE'S (GAO) DRAFT REPORT ENTITLED, "RYAN WHITE CARE ACT: IMPROVEMENTS NEEDED IN OVERSIGHT OF GRANTEES" (GAO-12-610)

Further, four of the 25 grantees said they were told that HRSA could not provide needed TA due to budget constraints, forcing the grantees to seek TA from other sources or using their own administrative funds.

HRSA provides a wide array of technical assistance and training services to grantees through a variety of strategic approaches and dissemination strategies. These include individualized and on-site peer and expert consultation, reverse site visits (where grantees meet with HAB staff in HRSA offices in Rockville, MD), national and regional meetings, consultative meetings and conferences, conference calls and webinars, development of products and training curricula in hard copy or web-based, email listservs, and other means of regular communications and information. Technical assistance is provided to clinical service providers, planning bodies, and other constituents to improve the performance of grantees. For example, through HAB's national technical assistance contract, during the last full year for which such information is available (FY 2010), there were 150 active technical assistance interventions of various types, many of which were for example, consultant on-site visits to grantees.

Between January 2010 and September 2011, the Technical Assistance Resources Guidance, Education, and Training (TARGET) Center, HAB's web-based resource for technical assistance, received 45,612 hits (3,801 per month). This website allows HAB, other federal partners, and grantees to efficiently share up-to-date valuable technical assistance resources and online training with each other.

However, in response to the view expressed by these four grantees, HRSA is strengthening its efforts to communicate the availability of technical assistance through the following actions: providing more information on the availability of technical assistance on its grantee listserv; reinforcing available technical assistance resources during monthly PO calls; National Association of State and Territorial AIDS Directors outreach to its membership and grantees; biweekly email to grantees; and posting more extensive information on the website on how to access technical assistance from HRSA.

HRSA makes decisions to prioritize technical assistance based on grantee need and program priorities. In FY 2012, HRSA invested approximately $14.5 million on Ryan White Program specific technical assistance, which includes substantive content on administration, policy, and fiscal management among other topics. For example, HRSA has a *Fiscal Management Cooperative Agreement*, which enlists a technical contractor to work with grantees to understand and effectively manage fiscal aspects of their programs.

4

**GENERAL COMMENTS OF THE DEPARTMENT OF HEALTH AND HUMAN
SERVICES (HHS) ON THE GOVERNMENT ACCOUNTABILITY OFFICE'S
(GAO) DRAFT REPORT ENTITLED, "RYAN WHITE CARE ACT:
IMPROVEMENTS NEEDED IN OVERSIGHT OF GRANTEES" (GAO-12-610)**

In addition, approximately $34 million was used to support clinical training via the
national AIDS Education Training Center program. Much like the needs assessment
process that a Ryan White HIV/AIDS Program grantee undertakes in identifying the need
for services, HAB engages in a formal process of assessing the need for training and
technical assistance, and the existence of current or other available resources, to
specifically identify technical assistance priorities, which includes extensive input from
grantees. At times, HRSA does recommend grantees utilize their Ryan White Program
funding for technical assistance after weighing competing priorities for HRSA's technical
assistance.

**"Three other grantees told us they turned to NASTAD for TA when HRSA could
not provide it or when PO responses to their questions were delayed."**

As GAO states in a footnote, HRSA has a cooperative agreement with NASTAD to
provide technical assistance to grantees. The partnership between HRSA and NASTAD
dates back to 1998. Therefore, the fact that the three grantees GAO interviewed turned to
NASTAD for technical assistance is consistent with HRSA's overall technical assistance
strategy. Depending on the particular need, POs would appropriately direct grantees to
this resource. Please see Appendix 2 for more detail on NASTAD's technical assistance
activities.

HRSA Did Not Prioritize Site Visits Strategically

GAO identified, through PO interviews, that site visits are a valuable and important form
of oversight. HAB uses a strategy for site visit selection based on risk analysis. GAO
notes that HRSA prioritizes site visits based on two elements: grantees without a recent
site visit and grantees with problems. GAO's definition of "grantees with problems" is
limited to a grantee that "had been placed on restrictive drawdown, had a relevant finding
in their annual single audit, or both from 2008 through 2011." However, GAO
acknowledges that HRSA officials stated there could be other indications of grantee
problems.

As an indication of grantee problems, HAB examines emergent and critical public health
and clinical challenges: fiscal and administrative challenges in a jurisdiction, grantee or
program; grantee non-compliance with statutory and programmatic requirements and
oversight; and technical assistance needs. This was the case with grantees in Puerto Rico
and the U.S. Virgin Islands (USVI), which had a long history of sustained fiscal and

5

**GENERAL COMMENTS OF THE DEPARTMENT OF HEALTH AND HUMAN
SERVICES (HHS) ON THE GOVERNMENT ACCOUNTABILITY OFFICE'S
(GAO) DRAFT REPORT ENTITLED, "RYAN WHITE CARE ACT:
IMPROVEMENTS NEEDED IN OVERSIGHT OF GRANTEES" (GAO-12-610)**

clinical challenges that were life-threatening to patients and had the potential to increase
incidence of HIV in those jurisdictions.[1]

Site visit priorities are reviewed quarterly and as needed by the PO, branch chief, division
director, and HAB associate administrator. POs outline their rationale for site visits in
quarterly travel plans, which include an explicit purpose for the visit. In addition,
leadership holds weekly meetings during which they discuss problem grantees and
mechanisms, including site visits, to address these problems. While HAB's site visit
strategy was not documented at the time of GAO's review, HAB will update its
Operations Manual to include more specific information about its strategy for site visit
selection. In addition, documentation of each of these steps will be included in the EHB.

Furthermore, GAO references the "Manual for Monitoring Grants and Cooperative
Agreements for Federal Personnel, which lists several "grant characteristics that should
be considered in selecting projects for on-site monitoring." "Cost and Total Support" is
one factor among many — including "Prior Indications of Problems." (See Appendix 3 for
this reference). In the report, GAO observed that "some of the grantees that HRSA
visited most during these four years had relatively small grant awards, indicating fewer
people being served by that grantee, which suggests that the agency did not prioritize site
visits based on grant funding level." GAO correctly notes that HRSA did not have grant
funding level as the primary factor in prioritizing site visits, nor is it a requirement.
While funding level is one factor, many large HRSA grantees, such as states, have
multiple internal controls in place. These controls help to make them less at risk for
problems than smaller grantees without such infrastructure.

The report specifically identifies visits to Puerto Rico and the USVI, which are
unfortunate examples of severe grantee problems. The USVI and Puerto Rico face
significant challenges in providing services to people living with HIV/AIDS and in
managing their Ryan White Program resources. The incidence and prevalence rates of
HIV and AIDS combined with fragile public health infrastructure commonly present
unique challenges in the territories and jurisdictions. The Caribbean has the second
highest regional HIV prevalence in the world after sub-Saharan Africa (Source: UNAIDS

---

[1] The situation in Puerto Rico for HIV/AIDS patients was so severe it was the subject of New York Times
front page story on June 5, 2007.
http://www.nytimes.com/2007/06/05/health/05puerto.html?ex=1338696000&en=5ca438412696d1bb&ei=5
088&partner=rssnyt&emc=rss The situation in the U.S. Virgin Islands for HIV/AIDs patients was so
severe it was the subject of an article in the VI Daily News, "VI Health Department's Failures Force
Patients to go without Drugs," 2/11/09.

6

**GENERAL COMMENTS OF THE DEPARTMENT OF HEALTH AND HUMAN
SERVICES (HHS) ON THE GOVERNMENT ACCOUNTABILITY OFFICE'S
(GAO) DRAFT REPORT ENTITLED, "RYAN WHITE CARE ACT:
IMPROVEMENTS NEEDED IN OVERSIGHT OF GRANTEES" (GAO-12-610)**

2011). Puerto Rico's HIV infection incidence rate is nearly twice that of the United
States, and their death rate is over three times higher. The USVI has an HIV infection rate
nearly three times as high as the US, and the rate of perinatal infected persons living with
HIV/AIDS in Puerto Rico is nearly three times the rate in the United States. These data
demonstrate the significant increased burden of HIV both medically and financially in
Puerto Rico compared to the U.S. overall.[2]

Both grantees have program implementation challenges that far exceed most other Ryan
White Program grantees. In Puerto Rico, HRSA identified longstanding and critical
issues in providing care to people living with HIV/AIDS including:

1. Disruptions in access to HIV medications and medical care;
2. Ongoing vacancies in key positions within the Ryan White Part A and B
   programs;
3. Inability to establish and execute contracts for HIV services; and
4. Difficulty complying with legislative requirements such as payor of last resort.

Through site visits, HRSA found that Part A and B contracts were not executed in a
timely manner causing hardships to patients. In addition, key staff vacancies prevented
appropriate oversight and monitoring of subcontractors and the ADAP was not managed
consistent with Ryan White Program's statutory payor of last resort requirement.

As the result of the close work between HRSA and Puerto Rico Part A and B program
staff, these issues have largely been resolved. However, Puerto Rico requires continued
close monitoring due to the high rate of key staff turnover.

---

[2] The Puerto Rico Department of Health reported a total of 34,912 AIDS cases as of June 3, 2011. The
Centers for Disease Control and Prevention (CDC) estimated the HIV infection incidence rate of 28.2 per
100,000 people in 2010 in Puerto Rico compared with a U.S. rate of 16.3 per 100,000 people. In Puerto
Rico, the death rate from HIV/AIDS was 10.9 per 100,000 people compared to the U.S. rate of 3.3 per
100,000 people (2008 data). In the USVI, the CDC estimated that in 2010 the HIV infection incidence rate
was 42.8 per 100,000 people compared to the U.S. rate of 16.3 people 100,000. The rate of perinatal
infected persons living with HIV/AIDS in the USVI is 19.1 per 100,000 people compared to the U.S. rate
of 9.1 per 100,000 people. The rate of perinatal infected persons in the USVI is 26.4 per 100,000 people
compared to the U.S. rate of 9.1 per 100,000 people.

7

**GENERAL COMMENTS OF THE DEPARTMENT OF HEALTH AND HUMAN
SERVICES (HHS) ON THE GOVERNMENT ACCOUNTABILITY OFFICE'S
(GAO) DRAFT REPORT ENTITLED, "RYAN WHITE CARE ACT:
IMPROVEMENTS NEEDED IN OVERSIGHT OF GRANTEES" (GAO-12-610)**

The Virgin Island Health Department also suffers from significant fiscal, administrative, infrastructure, and operational deficiencies. HAB has identified longstanding and critical issues in the USVI in providing care to people living with HIV/AIDS.

In FY 2008, the USVI grantee experienced significant fiscal and administrative issues, prompting HRSA to strongly urge the territory to select and utilize a fiscal agent for the administration of the grant, including payments to providers. The problems reached a breaking point in 2009, when HRSA found that HIV/AIDS medications were unavailable to HIV/AIDS infected patients, and the USVI's Ryan White AIDS Drug Assistance Programs had been closed. The absence of antiretroviral treatment creates a significant public health risk, particularly in HIV transmission rates in pregnant women to their unborn children. For example, in the United States, with antiretroviral treatment, mother-to-child transmission rates are less than three percent. Without antiretroviral treatment, mother-to-child transmission rates are at least 25 percent. In addition, intermittent access to antiretroviral medication can lead to antiretroviral drug resistance, which creates an additional serious public health concern. These circumstances required immediate Ryan White program efforts to restore access to ADAP drugs. Several site visits were made over a relatively short period of time to assess, plan, and assist in implementing significant efforts to reinstate access to medications and ensure that the problems leading to the closure of the ADAP were remedied.

In 2011, the grantee experienced significant staff turnover and changes in their fiduciary agent, which warranted direct assistance from the HRSA PO in the areas of fiscal administration and program management.

Site visit findings in the USVI have included: failure to execute contracts with the fiduciary/administrative agent in a timely manner; improperly used Ryan White Part B funds across grant years; lack of payments to Part B providers, including the fiduciary/administrative agent; failure to maintain adequate supply of HIV medications, leading to recurring shortages; late submission of their funding application; inability to account for how grant funds were expended for grant years; lack of adequate planning processes to provide HIV-related services for the HIV infected population; and staff vacancies preventing appropriate monitoring of subcontractors.

In response to site visit findings, through close work with HRSA, the USVI established a contract with a fiduciary/administrative agent to improve contracting processes; established an expedited payment process between the USVI and the

8

**GENERAL COMMENTS OF THE DEPARTMENT OF HEALTH AND HUMAN
SERVICES (HHS) ON THE GOVERNMENT ACCOUNTABILITY OFFICE'S
(GAO) DRAFT REPORT ENTITLED, "RYAN WHITE CARE ACT:
IMPROVEMENTS NEEDED IN OVERSIGHT OF GRANTEES" (GAO-12-610)**

fiduciary/administrative agent to pay subcontractors; developed a plan for addressing
medication shortages; received training at agencies involved in the fiscal, grants
management and procurement processes of the Ryan White Part B program; developed a
plan to deliver HIV-related services; received technical assistance on proper reporting of
expenditures; and received extensive technical assistance on sub-grantee monitoring.

At the time, because of the number of problems continually arising in the USVI, HRSA
considered permanently stationing a seasoned HIV/AIDS program expert on site.
However, it was concluded that the use of travel funds was more economical and equally
effective.

**"Furthermore, the District of Columbia, which received approximately $21 million
in 2011 CARE Act funding based on an estimated 17,250 living HIV/AIDS cases at
the end of 2009, had a history of problems and would require HRSA spend little in
travel funds to conduct site visits, but received only one visit over the four years."**

HRSA uses various tools and mechanisms to provide monitoring, oversight, and technical
assistance to grantees. GAO is accurate in noting that D.C. had only one comprehensive,
PO-led site visit over four years. However, in follow up to the site visit noted by GAO in
2008, HRSA met with the District of Columbia Department of Health to outline a
comprehensive 24-month technical assistance plan. In the subsequent four years, in
accordance with that plan, D.C. received over more than ten different interventions to
address both fiscal and grants management issues.

It is HRSA's practice to implement technical assistance and monitor the progress of the
grantee over the duration of technical assistance plans before conducting subsequent in-
depth diagnostic site visits. Consequently, meetings, email exchanges, phone calls to
review progress, and other interventions were held in both D.C. and HRSA's Rockville,
MD, offices to address its challenges directly. Additionally, in 2010 HRSA began
planning the D.C. Cross Part Clinical Quality Management Collaborative that was
implemented in 2011. Through this Collaborative partnership between HRSA and D.C.,
HRSA provides training and technical assistance to the Ryan White HIV/AIDS Program
grantees in the D.C. Eligible Metropolitan Area to improve quality of care and quality
improvement initiatives in their programs. While, as GAO notes, visits like these are not
documented as compliance or oversight monitoring visits, to date, this effort alone has
resulted in six separate technical assistance visits/trainings between January 2011 and
February 2012 and seven webinars between May 2011 and April 2012. As previously

9

**GENERAL COMMENTS OF THE DEPARTMENT OF HEALTH AND HUMAN
SERVICES (HHS) ON THE GOVERNMENT ACCOUNTABILITY OFFICE'S
(GAO) DRAFT REPORT ENTITLED, "RYAN WHITE CARE ACT:
IMPROVEMENTS NEEDED IN OVERSIGHT OF GRANTEES" (GAO-12-610)**

indicated, per GAO's recommendations, all interactions with grantees will be
documented in a centralized EHB and accessible to all relevant program and grants staff.

POs Did Not Always Review Annual Single Audit Findings:

The GAO draft report states that "Some POs" were not always aware of annual single
audit findings for their grantees. During the period of GAO's review, HRSA's Division
of Financial Integrity was informing HAB senior staff, who supervise POs, of single
audit findings related either to a monetary finding or a programmatic issue. The Division
Director or Branch Chief would then refer to POs any findings that required actions on
their part. In addition, when all of the audit findings have been satisfactorily resolved,
HRSA included a summary statement indicating this resolution in EHB as part of the
Financial Assessment.

However, in response to the GAO draft report, the Division of Financial Integrity will
communicate single audit findings directly to both POs and HAB Division Directors. As
of April 30, 2012, HRSA has included a detailed description of all audit findings, as well
as the corrective actions taken to address the findings, in EHB, which is fully accessible
to POs. Consistent with this new direction, DFI is now sending POs copies of the final
audit determination letter for every audit and a summary sheet detailing the findings and
corrective action taken.

**HRSA Did Not Clearly Communicate with Grantees about the Restrictive
Drawdown Process.**

Acknowledging the experiences of grantees interviewed by GAO, HRSA is strengthening
its process around grantee communication. As of May 1, 2012, HAB uses an improved
documentation process in the official file of actions related to drawdown restrictions.
The process includes enhancements for frequent communication to the grantees
indicating reasons for the restriction, how to request access to awarded funds, and how to
correct deficiencies. As of 2012, HRSA has modified the language on its "Notice of
Award," the official legal document of the grant agreement, to include the specific reason
for the drawdown restriction, how to request the funds, and notice on the process for
resolving the condition. HRSA can lift the restriction once the grantee addresses the
deficiencies.

HRSA will hold a webinar in June 2012 for Part A and Part B grantees to alert them to
these changes in the drawdown restriction process. Additional information, resources

10

<u>**GENERAL COMMENTS OF THE DEPARTMENT OF HEALTH AND HUMAN
SERVICES (HHS) ON THE GOVERNMENT ACCOUNTABILITY OFFICE'S
(GAO) DRAFT REPORT ENTITLED, "RYAN WHITE CARE ACT:
IMPROVEMENTS NEEDED IN OVERSIGHT OF GRANTEES" (GAO-12-610)**</u>

and examples will be provided on the Target Center website under the heading "Manage
Your Grant" which already provides tools and resources for grantee use and reference.
Additionally, all grantees currently on restricted drawdown (5 for Part A and 9 for Part B)
will be reviewed using HAB's newly refined process prior to the June 2012 conference
call. During this assessment, HAB's review will include the rationale for the condition,
the technical assistance offered, progress made by the grantee in addressing the reasons
for the condition, and improvement needed to address deficiencies. Using the above
information, HAB will document either a decision to lift the restriction or provide a clear
rationale for continuing the condition and necessary steps for addressing deficiencies.
Ryan White Part A and Part B Grantees remaining on restricted drawdown for FY 2013
will receive Notice of Awards with the new language and will be impacted by the new
process.

The procedures build improved frequency and quality of communication with the
grantees. HRSA will continue to provide related technical assistance via email and
phone, and more complete information will also be formally conveyed in the Notice of
Awards. In response to the GAO report, HRSA has instituted improved procedures to
ensure that this documentation will now all be included in the official grant file of the
EHB.

**HRSA Lack of Records and Changes in PO Assignments Further Challenge its
Oversight of CARE Act Grantees**

All government records are to be maintained according to record control schedules
outlined by the National Archives and Records Administration (NARA). HRSA is
required to follow these policies and may not retain records for a shorter or longer period
of time than the approved retention schedule. Consequently, files maintained by the PO,
may be disposed of sooner than the official grant file in accordance with the appropriate
schedule. At the time of the GAO review, HAB was operating under dated records
retention practices which, as GAO notes, could challenge oversight of grantees.

Prior to and during the GAO study, HRSA began reviewing its records management
program, including seeking approval of new record control schedules from NARA. In
December 2011, HRSA formed a workgroup on records management with program and
grant staff across the agency to streamline various retention schedules for program and
grant record retention practices. HRSA will be providing additional training and updated
policies for the HAB PO's and grants management specialists on the contents of the
official grant file.

11

**GENERAL COMMENTS OF THE DEPARTMENT OF HEALTH AND HUMAN
SERVICES (HHS) ON THE GOVERNMENT ACCOUNTABILITY OFFICE'S
(GAO) DRAFT REPORT ENTITLED, "RYAN WHITE CARE ACT:
IMPROVEMENTS NEEDED IN OVERSIGHT OF GRANTEES" (GAO-12-610)**

**HRSA Recently Issued National Standards for Grantee Monitoring of Service
Providers, but HRSA's Implementation Created Challenges for Grantees.**

In the report, GAO notes that seven grantees expressed particular concern about the
annual site visit requirement for service providers. Currently, the National Monitoring
Standards require an annual comprehensive monitoring site visit as delineated in Section
I.E. of the Part A and B Universal Standards. HRSA arrived at this annual site visit
decision based on previous OIG investigations that examined grantee and subgrantee
practices, e.g. its 2004 report, *"The Ryan White CARE Act Title I and Title II Grantees'
Monitoring of Subgrantees."* HRSA is currently working with the small number of
grantees that have expressed challenges with this requirement and is providing flexibility
that allows for oversight within the grantee's functional capacity.

12

GENERAL COMMENTS OF THE DEPARTMENT OF HEALTH AND HUMAN SERVICES (HHS) ON THE GOVERNMENT ACCOUNTABILITY OFFICE'S (GAO) DRAFT REPORT ENTITLED, "RYAN WHITE CARE ACT: IMPROVEMENTS NEEDED IN OVERSIGHT OF GRANTEES" (GAO-12-610)

Recommendations for Executive Action

Given the improvements over the past few years in creating a core foundation to support and strengthen overall program monitoring and oversight capacity of the Ryan White Program, coupled with a commitment to continually assess and improve on this foundation, the Department concurs with all five Recommendations for Executive Action (Page 40 of the draft report). HRSA is already in the process of planning and/or implementing many of these recommendations:

Ensure that the agency is implementing the key elements of grantee oversight consistent with HHS and HRSA guidance, including routine monitoring, the provision of technical assistance, site visits and restrictive drawdown.

Health and Human Services agrees with GAO. HRSA will continue working to improve its structures for monitoring and overseeing these grantees. We appreciate the recommendations that have been made on strategies for making improvements. HRSA is conducting the following activities to implement this recommendation:

Routine Monitoring:

HRSA's electronic grants monitoring system, the Electronic Handbook (EHB), will now consolidate and serve as the centralized location for all activity related to oversight and monitoring.

- The upgraded system will help Project Officers (POs) interact with grantees and document these interactions. Examples include improved uploading and organizing of project documentation and records analysis.
- The enhanced EHB will also include a new management tool to allow program officials to electronically track grantee monitoring activities, grantee data and reporting submissions, as well as other key information to ensure adequate oversight and program effectiveness. The tool also will allow tracking of the status of grant actions, grantee data and reporting submissions, and timeliness of completion of assigned PO and Branch Chief tasks based on established benchmarks. The EHB will make all information accessible to all HRSA staff with monitoring and oversight responsibilities (e.g., program and DFI staff).

13

GENERAL COMMENTS OF THE DEPARTMENT OF HEALTH AND HUMAN SERVICES (HHS) ON THE GOVERNMENT ACCOUNTABILITY OFFICE'S (GAO) DRAFT REPORT ENTITLED, "RYAN WHITE CARE ACT: IMPROVEMENTS NEEDED IN OVERSIGHT OF GRANTEES" (GAO-12-610)

- Routine monitoring calls and other communications with grantees, as well as the associated documentation, are tracked during biweekly supervision meetings between POs and Branch Chiefs. Until the upgraded EHB is fully functional, documentation will be posted on the HIV/AIDS Bureau's (HAB) internal team website after review by the Branch Chief. This assures that documentation is occurring and relevant information is accessible to all key staff.

Provision of Technical Assistance:

HAB is strengthening its efforts to communicate the availability of technical assistance through the following actions: providing more information on the availability of technical assistance on its grantee listserv; reinforcing available technical assistance resources during monthly PO calls; planning more National Association of State and Territorial AIDS Directors outreach to grantees; providing additional information for the HAB biweekly email to grantees; and posting more extensive information on the website on how to accessing technical assistance from HRSA.

Site Visits:

- HRSA has been working to leverage an existing site visit module, which was piloted by another HRSA program, and creating an agency-wide tool within the EHB to plan, schedule, track, and report site visits consistent with HRSA standards. This includes a site visit planning, execution, and report module that assures documentation in the electronic system.
- HRSA will leverage its regional network to improve grantee monitoring and oversight, which will be discussed in depth related to GAO's third recommendation.

Restrictive drawdown:

As of May 1, 2012, HRSA has implemented an improved procedure to record and document in the official file actions related to drawdown restrictions. The improved procedures also include enhancements to provide more standardized and frequent communication with the grantees on the reason for the restriction, how to request their funds, and how to address the deficiency. HRSA has also expanded the language on its Notice of Award to include the specific reason for the drawdown restriction, how to request the funds, and notice on the process for resolving the condition.

14

<u>**GENERAL COMMENTS OF THE DEPARTMENT OF HEALTH AND HUMAN
SERVICES (HHS) ON THE GOVERNMENT ACCOUNTABILITY OFFICE'S
(GAO) DRAFT REPORT ENTITLED, "RYAN WHITE CARE ACT:
IMPROVEMENTS NEEDED IN OVERSIGHT OF GRANTEES" (GAO-12-610)**</u>

Going forward, HRSA will ensure that this process is keeping grantees fully informed
while minimizing any unnecessary administrative burden on the grantees. Beginning
with the FY 2013 Part A and Part B awards, HRSA's Office of Federal Assistance
Management, along with HAB leadership and POs, will conduct annual reviews of these
restrictions as part of the annual award cycle. Through this additional team based
oversight, HRSA will examine the following for each grantee on drawdown:

- The length of time the grantee has been on drawdown;
- The technical assistance provided to date to help address the deficiency; and
- Whether the grantee is making progress in addressing the deficiency.

Using the above information, HRSA will document either a decision to lift the restriction
or to provide additional technical assistance to the grantee. Additionally, the decision to
lift the restriction can continue to be made throughout the year, whenever the deficiency
has been addressed.

<u>Training</u>:

Training of POs and managers is a critical part of improvement work in these four areas
of grantee oversight. HRSA established the HRSA Learning Institute (HLI) in 2010 to
better meet and standardize the training and development needs of HRSA POs. In June
2010, HLI conducted an agency-wide training and development needs assessment to help
further assess and clarify PO training and development needs. Since that time, HLI has
implemented a number of courses for POs.

Most recently, HAB has developed a competency-based HAB Project Officer Core
Technical curriculum to ensure that all POs are proficient to meet the mission of HAB.
Developed in December 2011, and now being implemented, HAB uses a curriculum that
formalizes and expands on the trainings that had been offered previously. The curriculum
focuses on identifying the critical technical competencies for POs in performing their
roles and responsibilities. The HAB competency-based curriculum includes learning
modules that focus on specific technical skills of HAB POs. The learning modules in the
HAB PO curriculum support the HAB technical competencies that set the HRSA/HAB's
expectations for the knowledge, skills and behaviors needed for the roles and functions
performed at HAB. Please see Appendix 4 for the complete description of the HAB PO
Core Technical Curriculum. To ensure the policies and procedures covered in these
courses are being followed, POs will meet with their supervisors on a biweekly basis to
assess and reinforce appropriate grantee monitoring.

15

<u>GENERAL COMMENTS OF THE DEPARTMENT OF HEALTH AND HUMAN
SERVICES (HHS) ON THE GOVERNMENT ACCOUNTABILITY OFFICE'S
(GAO) DRAFT REPORT ENTITLED, "RYAN WHITE CARE ACT:
IMPROVEMENTS NEEDED IN OVERSIGHT OF GRANTEES" (GAO-12-610)</u>

<u>Assess and revise its record retention management program so that complete
grantee files are available for a period of time that HRSA determines will satisfy all
of the agency's grantee oversight needs.</u>

In December 2011, HRSA began a comprehensive review and assessment of its current
and previously approved records retention schedule. Updates to that schedule will be
completed and submitted to the National Archives and Records Administration (NARA)
for approval this year. Once approved by NARA, HRSA will publish the updated
schedule and provide training to all project officers on its application. In the interim,
HRSA has formed an Agency wide workgroup on records management with program and
grant staff across the Agency to review and where needed, strengthen policies and
procedures for program and grant record retention practices.

Lastly, in 2012, HRSA is offering training to POs and grants management specialists
beyond the traditional scope of training that will focus on further strengthening their
records management responsibilities.

<u>Develop a strategic, risk-based approach for selecting grantees for site visits that
better targets the use of available resources to ensure that HRSA visits grantees at
regular and timely intervals.</u>

The HRSA Program Integrity Initiative was launched in June 2010 with an objective of
identifying and targeting the greatest risks, reducing those risks through new or enhanced
oversight activities, and identifying and sharing new and best practices. HRSA's
underlying principle is to work to fully integrate program integrity elements into daily
operations. The Initiative combines the existing internal HRSA integrity activities related
to internal controls, compliance with laws and regulations, and prevention of improper
payments, with a focus on enhancing external integrity activities associated with HRSA
grantees. The Administrator sent to each HRSA employee in December of 2010, and to
each HRSA grantee in January 2011, a letter stressing the importance of program
integrity and describing the new and enhanced HRSA integrity activities.

The HRSA Initiative began with the establishment of a prioritized agenda for program
integrity activities. These priorities and actions to date are described below.

16

**GENERAL COMMENTS OF THE DEPARTMENT OF HEALTH AND HUMAN
SERVICES (HHS) ON THE GOVERNMENT ACCOUNTABILITY OFFICE'S
(GAO) DRAFT REPORT ENTITLED, "RYAN WHITE CARE ACT:
IMPROVEMENTS NEEDED IN OVERSIGHT OF GRANTEES" (GAO-12-610)**

1. Provide program integrity staff dedicated to addressing specific grantee issues

Beginning in early FY 2011, HRSA increased program integrity staffing, both at HRSA's
headquarters and in HRSA's ten regional offices, to support the agency in its monitoring
and delivery of financial and technical support to grantees. These regional program
integrity analysts, in addition to HAB staff, will conduct site visits as needed to monitor
grantee performance, provide technical assistance and support, and when appropriate,
develop and monitor corrective action plans.

**2. Increase HRSA's capacity to perform grantee financial reviews and other grants
management functions**

As noted earlier, HRSA is updating its electronic grants monitoring system, Electronic
Handbook (EHB), to be the central location for all oversight and monitoring
documentation, including standardized site visiting elements. This will allow program
and grants oversight leadership to conduct deeper analyses by program, geographic
location, and grantees across and within HRSA programs. Specifically, the site visit tool
will provide an enterprise risk-based approach for planning, prioritizing, scheduling,
tracking and reporting site visits. Further, in response to the GAO recommendation for a
centralized repository of Ryan White grantee site visits, an accessible electronic
infrastructure will be completed and populated by September 2012.

3. Improve site visits through improved tools and analysis

The HRSA Program Integrity Workgroup serves as an information clearinghouse on site
visit procedures to gain knowledge of the current best practices of each organization.
Additionally, HRSA has undertaken data mining activities which are being used to
identify potential issues, risks, and anomalies that may indicate a need for further analysis
and review.

Update and maintain a program manual for grantees

While HRSA has maintained updated program information on its website, HRSA
acknowledges the utility for grantees to have one consolidated program manual.
Therefore, HRSA will produce a printed Part A Manual, Part B Manual, and ADAP
Manual. The ADAP Manual, Part A and Part B Manuals will be available by the end of
calendar year 2012. When completed, these manuals will be made available on the
HRSA website. Grantees will be informed of the availability of the updated manuals and

17

GENERAL COMMENTS OF THE DEPARTMENT OF HEALTH AND HUMAN SERVICES (HHS) ON THE GOVERNMENT ACCOUNTABILITY OFFICE'S (GAO) DRAFT REPORT ENTITLED, "RYAN WHITE CARE ACT: IMPROVEMENTS NEEDED IN OVERSIGHT OF GRANTEES" (GAO-12-610)

training will be provided. Electronic versions will allow grantees on-line access and the ability to save, download and print as many copies as needed.

In the meantime, updated web-based resources have been and continue to be available on the HRSA website (e.g., contact list of grantees, legislative language, policies, AIDSInfo information on antiretrovirals, data-related resources for the RSR, eHandbook), which provide access to new information frequently used by Ryan White Program grantees. Additional efforts will be made to disseminate this information to grantees via email from POs, during monthly monitoring calls, program listservs, National Association of State and Territorial AIDS Directors' communications and products, HAB biweekly email, and postings on the Target Center.

Use the results of HRSA's survey of grantees to identify grantee training needs to allow them to comply with the National Monitoring Standards.

In addition to using other mechanisms for obtaining information on grantee training needs, HRSA implemented a grantee satisfaction survey in April 2012. Over the next year, these data will be used to evaluate opportunities for improvements, including the development of new resources for the grantee community. HRSA will provide feedback to grantees on the results of the survey and action taken. HRSA plans to repeat the survey annually to obtain ongoing assessment of Ryan White grantee needs.

As part of that restructuring, a new section, "Manage Your Ryan White Grant," was added in response to grantee requests for "one-stop shopping." Included in that section are comprehensive program manuals for Part A and Part B, which are updated as needed. HRSA also maintains an aggressive link management program to ensure integrity across the site. The entire site is scanned monthly and all broken links reported are either replaced with vetted and tested links or deleted within one week.

Within the year, HRSA will conduct a review of HAB's website, focusing on further improvements to make the site more accessible and useful. Specifically, HRSA will explore ways to:

- Enhance the grantee resource section of the website to minimize the number of links needed to arrive at program requirements;
- Enhance resource documents (including the National Monitoring Standards and Frequently Asked Questions) by including additional models of how to apply requirements or use resources;

18

<u>**GENERAL COMMENTS OF THE DEPARTMENT OF HEALTH AND HUMAN
SERVICES (HHS) ON THE GOVERNMENT ACCOUNTABILITY OFFICE'S
(GAO) DRAFT REPORT ENTITLED, "RYAN WHITE CARE ACT:
IMPROVEMENTS NEEDED IN OVERSIGHT OF GRANTEES" (GAO-12-610)**</u>

- Update the National Monitoring Standards documents so that grantees and
  subgrantees can directly link (electronically) to source citations for each
  requirement; and
- Create a grantee peer to peer portal and/or list-serve to encourage open
  communication and provide an e-site place to seek assistance and best practices
  for grant implementation.

19

**GENERAL COMMENTS OF THE DEPARTMENT OF HEALTH AND HUMAN
SERVICES (HHS) ON THE GOVERNMENT ACCOUNTABILITY OFFICE'S (GAO)
DRAFT REPORT ENTITLED, "RYAN WHITE CARE ACT: IMPROVEMENTS
NEEDED IN OVERSIGHT OF GRANTEES" (GAO-12-610)**

APPENDIX 1

Acquired Immune Deficiency Syndrome (AIDS) first appeared in the United States around 1969.
Doctors in Los Angeles, New York and San Francisco treated young gay men for Kaposi's
Sarcoma, a disease seen mostly in elderly Mediterranean men. In fact, the disease was named
"Gay Related Immune Deficiency." As time passed, the disease appeared in blood transfusion
patients, IV drug users, heterosexuals, bisexuals, and even new born babies. Consequently, the
Centers for Disease Control renamed the disease AIDS in 1982.

To provide resources for the care and treatment of people living with HIV, Congress passed the
Ryan White Comprehensive AIDS Resources Emergency (CARE) Act in 1990; the first grants
were distributed in 1991. In the two decades since then, the Act has been reauthorized four times.
From the beginning, the Ryan White HIV/AIDS Program has not been an entitlement program
like Medicaid and Medicare. Instead, the program is a discretionary budget item that funds, as
the payor of last resort:

- Part A grants to eligible metropolitan areas and transitional grant areas;
- Part B grants to U.S. States and territories; and
- Part C, D, and F grants directly to organizations.

The 1996 Act ensured access to highly active antiretroviral therapy through the AIDS Drug
Assistance Program funding. The 2000 reauthorization continued this tradition and expanded the
aims of the Ryan White HIV/AIDS Program by targeting infected individuals not in care by
providing funds for technical assistance and key points of entry into the medical system. The
reauthorization in 2006 sought to mitigate the high impact of the disease on African-American
and other minority communities by codifying the minority AIDS Initiative in the legislation.
Moreover, the reauthorization placed increased emphasis on medical care treatment. The 2009
reauthorization created new incentives to find HIV-infected persons and link them with primary
care.

Initially, AIDS was a death sentence. Today, the advancement of antiretroviral therapy has
changed the HIV/AIDS from an emergent disease to a manageable, chronic disease. The Ryan
White HIV/AIDS Program funds health provider training, medical care, treatment, referrals, and
social services to people living with HIV and AIDS in the United States, District of Columbia,
Puerto Rico, and U.S. Territories.

The change from an emergent disease to a chronic disease is not the only change. The "face" of
the HIV/AIDS epidemic has changed as well. Initially, the "face" of HIV/AIDS was young, gay

GENERAL COMMENTS OF THE DEPARTMENT OF HEALTH AND HUMAN SERVICES (HHS) ON THE GOVERNMENT ACCOUNTABILITY OFFICE'S (GAO) DRAFT REPORT ENTITLED, "RYAN WHITE CARE ACT: IMPROVEMENTS NEEDED IN OVERSIGHT OF GRANTEES" (GAO-12-610)

white men; today the "face" of HIV/AIDS is African American men and women, located primarily in the Southern portion of the United States. The Ryan White HIV/AIDS Program reaches those most in need- an estimated 73 percent racial minorities, 32 percent women, and 89 percent uninsured, underinsured and/or receiving public health benefits.

Ryan White HIV/AIDS Program accomplishments include:

- Funded programs to provide care, treatment and support services to approximately half of the people living with HIV/AIDS in the United States. Specifically, the Ryan White HIV/AIDS Program has served over 529,000 uninsured and underinsured of the 1.1 million people living with HIV/AIDs in the United States;
- Built networks and systems of care between public and private providers for a comprehensive response to the epidemic; and
- Extended the knowledge base and expertise to improve the quality of HIV/AIDS care and treatment across the health care system.

The HIV/AIDS Bureau works in partnership with Ryan White HIV/AIDS Program grantees to ensure compliance with statutory provisions. Moreover, the Bureau provides guidance, oversight and technical assistance to ensure that grantees receive the funds needed to serve people living with HIV/AIDS. If the grantees do not receive the funds, people living with HIV/AIDS will not receive needed primary care and medication therapy. The HIV/AIDS Bureau is fully committed to monitoring its grantees for compliance with the law.

GENERAL COMMENTS OF THE DEPARTMENT OF HEALTH AND HUMAN SERVICES (HHS) ON THE
GOVERNMENT ACCOUNTABILITY OFFICE'S (GAO) DRAFT REPORT ENTITLED, "RYAN WHITE CARE ACT:
IMPROVEMENTS NEEDED IN OVERSIGHT OF GRANTEES" (GAO-12-610)

APPENDIX 2

Technical Assistance Offered Through HRSA's ADAP Crisis Task Force and Structural Identified by HRSA's AIDS Drug Assistance Program (ADAP)

Date Range	Category of TA, Description
2008 – 2011	Arranged 15 peer-to-peer Technical Assistance Visits so that a more experienced ADAP could assist an ADAP with similar systems to improve clinical, fiscal, and programmatic and data management systems. The list of completed TA events is available.
2008 – 2011	8 ADAP All Member Conference Calls (2 per year)
2008 – 2011	52 Listserv alerts and bulletins in response to emergent, time-sensitive issues.
2008 – 2011	47 Individual ADAP telephone consultations (about 1 per month or 12 per yr). Produce written summaries of each call.
2008 – 2011	48 ADAP Clinical Management Newsletter.
2008	Emergency Preparedness Guide for ADAPs.
2009	Series of 3 briefs to address ADAP Cost Containment Strategies.
2010	Series of 6 multi-media tutorials on Implementing Quality Management Program for ADAPs.
May 8, 2012	Convened consultation meeting to develop a common application form for ADAP clients needing to access Patient Assistant Programs.
April 17-18, 2012	Convened consultation meeting to develop an adaptable financial forecasting tool for ADAPs.
April 17-18, 2012	In collaboration with the HRSA HAB data TA provider and HRSA/HAB developed implementation plan for ADAPs to initiate client level data collection and reporting, ensuring accurate data submission to HRSA/HAB.

GENERAL COMMENTS OF THE DEPARTMENT OF HEALTH AND HUMAN SERVICES (HHS) ON THE GOVERNMENT ACCOUNTABILITY OFFICES'S (GAO) DRAFT REPORT ENTITLED: "RYAN WHITE CARE ACT: IMPROVEMENTS NEEDED IN OVERSIGHT OF GRANTEES" (GAO-12-610)

Appendix 3

CHAPTER 6

Site Visits

Learning Objectives

After completing this chapter, you should be able to:

6.1 Identify factors to consider when selecting grants for site visits.

6.2 Explain previsit activities to perform to prepare both federal officials and recipient staff for a site visit.

6.3 Review recipient records and complete a site visit data collection checklist.

6.4 Evaluate a site visit report.

6.1 Selecting Projects for Onsite Monitoring

Site visits are particularly appropriate for complex or troublesome projects with special significance. Listed below are some grant characteristics that should be considered in selecting projects for onsite monitoring:

1. **Cost and Total Support.** Recipients with high-cost projects or with high composite levels of support from several different funding authorities within an agency may require closer monitoring.

2. **Complexity.** A project with multiple objectives or one involving experimental research techniques are examples of complex projects.

3. **Age of Program.** A new program, or one whose legislation has recently undergone substantial change, may require closer scrutiny than a long-established program.

4. **Prior Indications of Problems.** Available audit or evaluation findings, recipient requests for assistance, or data on the financial stability of an organization, may indicate a need for close monitoring.

Monitoring Grants and Cooperative Agreements for Federal Personnel

5. **Experience of Recipient.** A new or unstable organization, one receiving federal grants for the first time, or one with inexperienced key personnel may require close monitoring as well as technical assistance.

6. **Length of Grant.** A multi-year award, particularly one up for continuation funding, may require closer monitoring than a single year grant. Continuation awards that have never been visited may take precedence over new ones.

7. **Time Since Last Visit.** Recipients that have not been recently or previously visited may have priority for site visits.

8. **Geographic Location.** Proximity to other recipients scheduled for monitoring, or accessibility to the responsible program office, may make visits to certain sites more cost effective than others.

9. **Agency Priority.** Projects of high visibility/priority within the agency — and of high interest to Congress, the executive branch, or the public — may be given priority for site visits.

10. **Potential for Dissemination.** Projects that show potential for developing exemplary practices suitable for dissemination may be candidates for site visits.

Site visits can take several forms and be called for various reasons. **Traditional site visits** occur on a periodic basis for all or a sampling of a program's recipients. **New recipient site visits** take a proactive approach by assisting new recipients in ensuring that their systems meet the requirements for federal funds management and for the program under which they are receiving funds. **Reverse site visits** are used when the agency personnel have little or no funds for traveling, but travel funds can be built into recipients' budgets for a trip to the agency's office. These visits are sometimes scheduled concurrently so the agency can provide training for a group of recipients around the same time as their site visit meeting. **Reactive site visits** may be called when problems are noted, either through report review, a whistleblower complaint, or a recipient request for assistance.

GENERAL COMMENTS OF THE DEPARTMENT OF HEALTH AND HUMAN SERVICES (HHS) ON THE GOVERNMENT ACCOUNTABILITY OFFICE'S (GAO) DRAFT REPORT ENTITLED, "RYAN WHITE CARE ACT: IMPROVEMENTS NEEDED IN OVERSIGHT OF GRANTEES" (GAO-12-610)

APPENDIX 4

HIV/AIDS BUREAU (HAB)
PROJECT OFFICER CORE TECHNICAL CURRICULUM

Course or Topics/ Objectives	Competency Key Behaviors
HIV/AIDS 101: Care and Treatment **HIV/AIDS 201L PHS Guidelines for HIV Care and Treatment- Transferring Science into Practice**	Appreciate the foundations of public health and the significance of public health service. Demonstrate an understanding of HIV disease and applies that knowledge to the work of HAB in solving problems and implementing solutions.
Ryan White HIV/AIDS Programs • Overview of Parts A-F • Grant cycle from the Funding Opportunity Announcement (FOA) to closeout. • Roles of Division of Grants Management Operations (DGMO), the Office of General Counsel (OGC) and Division of Financial Integrity (DFI) in the management and administration of grant programs.	Describe how the Ryan White legislation is implemented and be able to use this knowledge in reviewing, monitoring and providing technical assistance to grant recipients. Explain the relationship of HAB with and the role of other government agencies in monitoring and administering the Ryan White HIV/AIDS legislative programs.
HAB Budget Process and Timeline **Roles and Responsibilities of HAB Project Officers** • Describe the roles and responsibilities of the HAB Project Officer • Apply the tools and resources available to monitor grantee performance and compliance • Provide guidance to grantees to the available technical assistance appropriate to meet grantee needs • Facilitate effective and timely communication with grantees • Analyze the various reports required from grantees to ensure grantee compliance with legislative, fiscal and programmatic requirements **Technical Assistance (TA) Tools and Resources: How to process requests for TA** • Describe the various technical assistance tools and resources available to grantees • Follow the appropriate processes and procedures for procuring technical assistance **Funding Opportunity Announcement (FOA) Review Process**	Adheres to Bureau/Division/Office established policies, processes and procedures Performs the specific roles and responsibilities identified for HAB Project Officers.
HAB Grant Application Process • Describe the grant application process, various funding opportunities and the limitations of the funding opportunities. • Explain how grants are funded, listed, submitted, processed and approved and approved (or disapproved). • Describe Application Review Process. • Explain the Notice of Award (NOA) to grantees. • Apply the program legislative regulation, policy, and guidance to effectively inform grantees	Ensures that grant applicants follow and adhere the grant application process established by the HRSA/HAB Evaluates and make recommendations on grant applications Effectively communicates the program legislative regulation, policy and guidance to grantees and partners concerning program priorities and objectives, the grant application process, NOA and the limitations of funding opportunities.

GENERAL COMMENTS OF THE DEPARTMENT OF HEALTH AND HUMAN SERVICES (HHS) ON THE
GOVERNMENT ACCOUNTABILITY OFFICE'S (GAO) DRAFT REPORT ENTITLED, "RYAN WHITE CARE ACT:
IMPROVEMENTS NEEDED IN OVERSIGHT OF GRANTEES" (GAO-12-610)

and partners about program priorities and objectives.	
Grantee Administrative Assessment and Monitoring • Discuss the framework and premise of the National Monitoring Standards for Grantee Monitoring Service Providers and how to help RW grantees meet federal requirements for program and fiscal management, monitoring and reporting • Use site visits, analyses or reports and other monitoring tools to evaluate grantee performance • Follow the site visit protocol established by HAB to include the type of site visit and the reporting requirements at the completion of the site visit • Compile and synthesize analyses of findings to determine performance improvement options • Make recommendations to achieve compliance and project goals • Explain the reasons for recommending drawdown restrictions for grantees • Describe the process for placing and removing drawdown restrictions on a grantee • Offer training and technical assistance to assist grantees in attaining compliance and improving operations	Evaluate grantee performance and make recommendations to achieve HRSA/HAB compliance and project goals. Analyze and synthesize evaluation results and use results to make recommendations for improvements in grantee performance or program implementation. Compile and synthesize analyses of findings to determine performance improvement options.
Foundation Course "Quality Improvement for public health practitioners" by Public Health Foundation. http://www.phf.org/quickguide/ContentPanel.aspx) • HAB Quality 101 course (existing HAB content) • HAB Quality 201 course (existing HAB content) • Performance Measures • Data Quality	Ability to maintain clinical quality management expectations and be knowledgeable of systems used. Ability to apply program management practices to routine work.
Financial Management for Project Officers • Describe the basic nonprofit financial management and accounting concepts • Differentiate different types of audits, auditing objectives, and audit opinions • Describe the role of the auditor • Interpret an Audit Report • Explain financial solvency • Describe the seven warning signs of potential fraud • Describe common schemes and their symptoms	Perform grantee budget reviews in terms of overall financial stability and risk factors. When problems in grantee financial management are discovered, monitor activity, confer with grantees and make referrals for intensive assistance or enforcement, as needed. Conduct regular reviews of grantee financial procedures and records, as well as program financial activities, to ensure compliance with requirements. Ensure that all grantee financial documentation is timely, clear, complete and accurate.
Data Utilization http://www.careacttarget.org/dataacademy/ • Introduction to Data utilization • RSR Data Training	Evaluate and integrate data and information that support decision-making and work flow within and across the settings where Ryan White HIV/AIDS Program services are delivered.
Introduction to Grants and Cooperative Agreements for Federal Personnel • Identify who is responsible at key stages during the grants process • Discuss the legal authorities governing federal assistance programs	Perform grantee budget reviews in terms of overall financial stability and risk factors. When problems in grantee financial management are

GENERAL COMMENTS OF THE DEPARTMENT OF HEALTH AND HUMAN SERVICES (HHS) ON THE GOVERNMENT ACCOUNTABILITY OFFICE'S (GAO) DRAFT REPORT ENTITLED, "RYAN WHITE CARE ACT: IMPROVEMENTS NEEDED IN OVERSIGHT OF GRANTEES" (GAO-12-610)

• Review the government wide program announcement template • Explore the technical review process for applications • Negotiate terms and conditions on a hypothetical grant Practice providing technical assistance on post award administrative requirements • Discuss audit requirements applicable to recipients of federal funds • Determine the appropriate course of action at the end of the grant period	discovered, monitor activity, confer with grantees and make referrals for intensive assistance or enforcement, as needed. Conduct regular reviews of grantee financial procedures and records, as well as program financial activities, to ensure compliance with requirements. Ensure that all grantee financial documentation is timely, clear, complete and accurate.
Monitoring Grants and Cooperative Agreements for Federal Personnel	
Cost Principles:2 CFR Part 220, 225, and 230 and FAR 31.2 (HRSA)	
EHB 101 • Navigate the electronic Hand Book (EHB) • Load and access documents and files in the EHB • Utilize the major functionalities in EHB to manage HRSA's grant portfolio such as project tracking, electronic funding memo process, conditions tracking and various reports • Become familiar with other essential documents and their retention requirements	Navigate the electronic Hand Book (EHB). Load and access documents and files in the EHB. Is familiar with other essential documents and their retention requirements.
Appropriations Law Seminar • Determine the legal availability of appropriations (including food, gifts, awards, taxes, and clothing) as to purpose, time, and amount • Promote the legal obligation of funds • Ensure that obligations are charged to the correct fund sources • Avoid violations of the Anti-deficiency Act (ADA)	Apply the knowledge for approaching appropriations issues that include the availability of appropriations as to purpose, amount and time, the necessary expense rule, the Anti-deficiency Act, augmentation, the bona fide needs rule, and multiyear contracting. Promote the legal obligation of funds. Ensure that obligations are charged to the correct fund sources.

Appendix IV: GAO Contact and Staff Acknowledgments

GAO Contact	Marcia Crosse, (202) 512-7114 or crossem@gao.gov
Acknowledgments	In addition to the contact named above, key contributors to this report were Tom Conahan, Assistant Director; Romonda Bumpus; Cathleen Hamann; Kathryn Richter; Sara Rudow; and Jennifer Whitworth.

GAO's Mission	The Government Accountability Office, the audit, evaluation, and investigative arm of Congress, exists to support Congress in meeting its constitutional responsibilities and to help improve the performance and accountability of the federal government for the American people. GAO examines the use of public funds; evaluates federal programs and policies; and provides analyses, recommendations, and other assistance to help Congress make informed oversight, policy, and funding decisions. GAO's commitment to good government is reflected in its core values of accountability, integrity, and reliability.
Obtaining Copies of GAO Reports and Testimony	The fastest and easiest way to obtain copies of GAO documents at no cost is through GAO's website (www.gao.gov). Each weekday afternoon, GAO posts on its website newly released reports, testimony, and correspondence. To have GAO e-mail you a list of newly posted products, go to www.gao.gov and select "E-mail Updates."
Order by Phone	The price of each GAO publication reflects GAO's actual cost of production and distribution and depends on the number of pages in the publication and whether the publication is printed in color or black and white. Pricing and ordering information is posted on GAO's website, http://www.gao.gov/ordering.htm. Place orders by calling (202) 512-6000, toll free (866) 801-7077, or TDD (202) 512-2537. Orders may be paid for using American Express, Discover Card, MasterCard, Visa, check, or money order. Call for additional information.
Connect with GAO	Connect with GAO on Facebook, Flickr, Twitter, and YouTube. Subscribe to our RSS Feeds or E-mail Updates. Listen to our Podcasts. Visit GAO on the web at www.gao.gov.
To Report Fraud, Waste, and Abuse in Federal Programs	Contact: Website: www.gao.gov/fraudnet/fraudnet.htm E-mail: fraudnet@gao.gov Automated answering system: (800) 424-5454 or (202) 512-7470
Congressional Relations	Katherine Siggerud, Managing Director, siggerudk@gao.gov, (202) 512-4400, U.S. Government Accountability Office, 441 G Street NW, Room 7125, Washington, DC 20548
Public Affairs	Chuck Young, Managing Director, youngc1@gao.gov, (202) 512-4800 U.S. Government Accountability Office, 441 G Street NW, Room 7149 Washington, DC 20548

www.ingramcontent.com/pod-product-compliance
Lightning Source LLC
Chambersburg PA
CBHW081136290526
45795CB00006B/2254